FERMENT

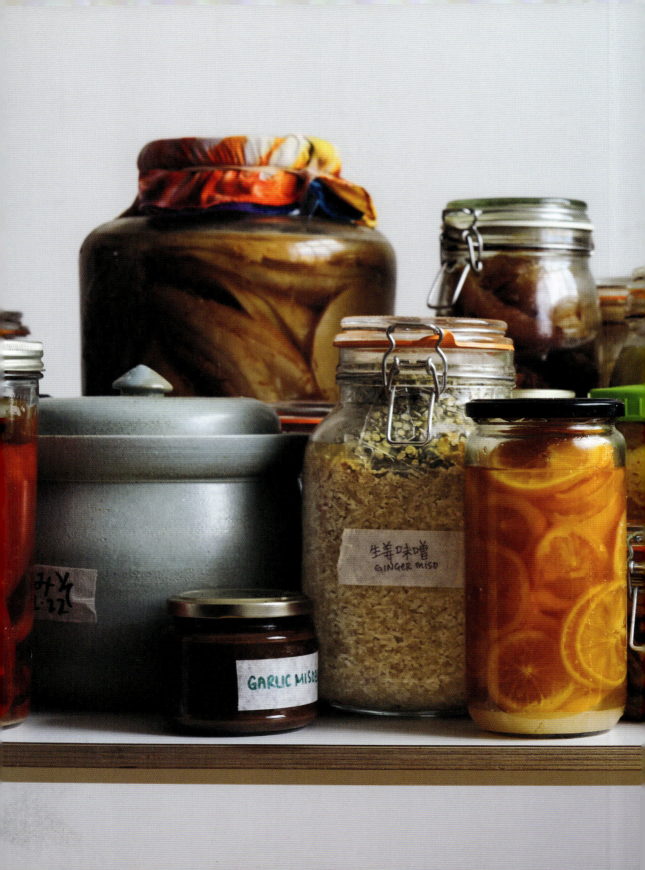

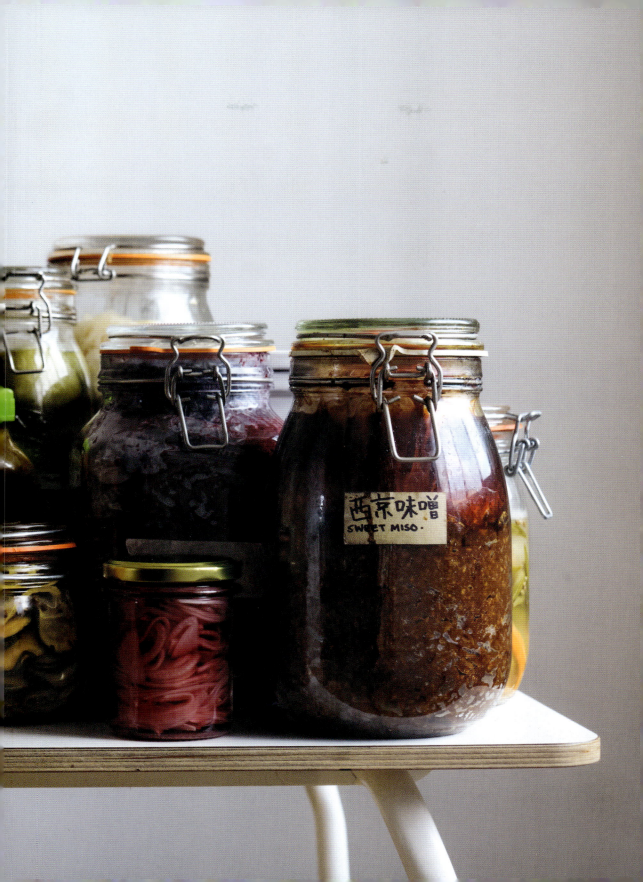

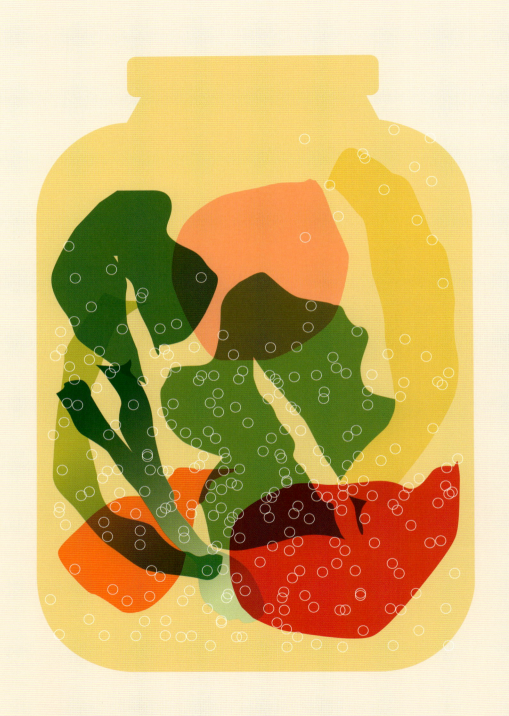

FERMENT

Simple Recipes from
My Multicultural Kitchen

Kenji Morimoto

NEW YORK

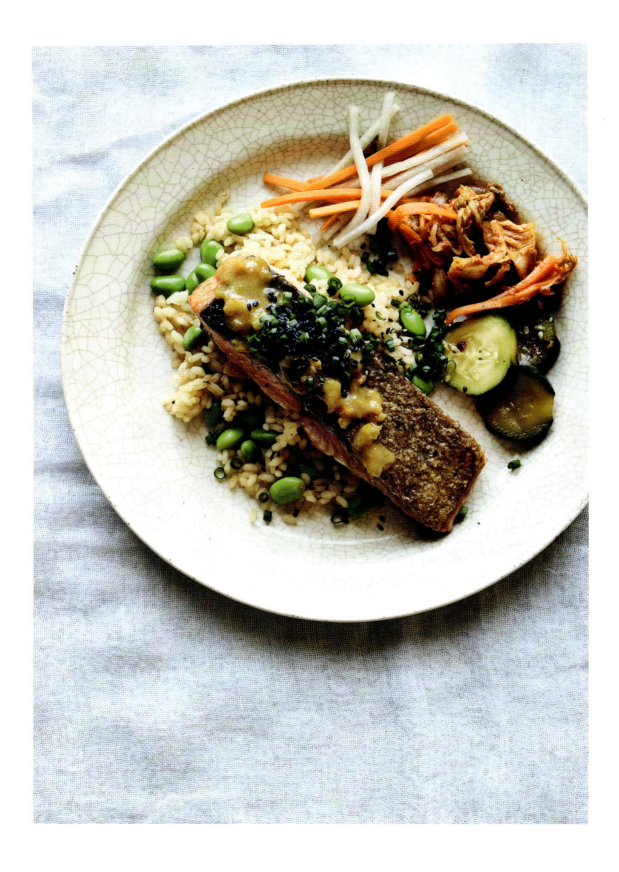

CONTENTS

INTRODUCTION	9
Preservation 101	14

FERMENTS 24

Lactofermentation	26
Kimchi	52
Miso	80
Pickling	106
Kombucha	124
Cheong	142

RECIPES 148

How to cook with pickles & ferments	150
Starters	152
Mains	188
Desserts	236
Cocktails	254

Acknowledgments	262
Index	264
About Kenji	270

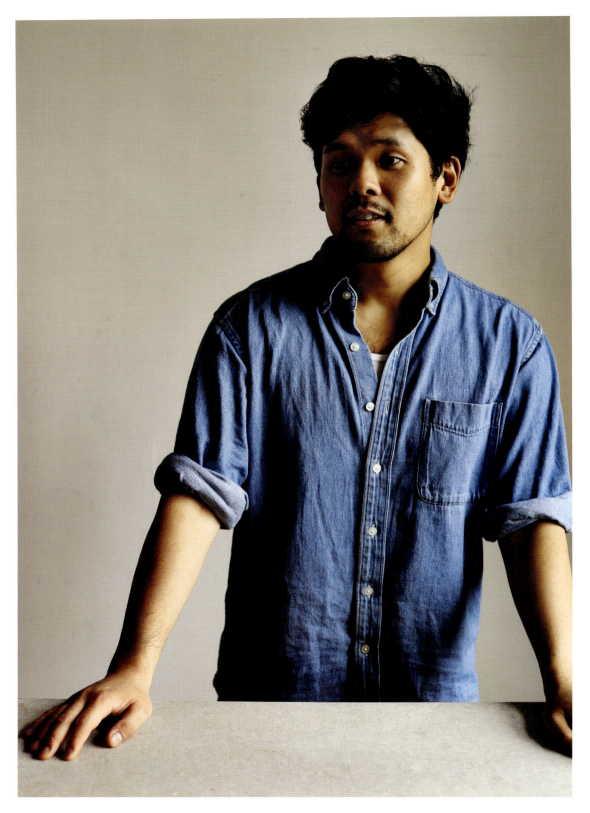

INTRODUCTION

Ferment is my simple guide to modern, everyday preservation techniques with which I connect diasporic dots and traditions within my home kitchen. Everything in these pages is easy to adapt based on what's in season or what's lingering in your fridge. My aim is that you feel empowered to preserve, ferment, and pickle with confidence, and learn how to use these results in your cooking. Flavorful, vibrant, and reflecting my global background, all of my recipes will showcase your creations and reinforce the versatility of preserving.

The kitchen was the center of my family's universe. Each person had a specific role, an unspoken understanding of process and duty which from afar appeared as a carefully choreographed routine. And as a child, I was in charge of making pickles.

Truth be told, this was one of the food items not claimed by grandparents or aunts and uncles for our often-elaborate meals, tables filled to the brim with dishes representing my family and our immigrant story. Pickle-making made sense for a young child. It was tactile in approach, encompassed endless creativity in vegetable and flavor combinations, and was magical in its transformative process. So I was immediately drawn to it.

I was a precocious kid, occasionally known to wear a white chef's hat and make complex dinners out of fairly bizarre ingredients (ask my parents about the elaborate multi-course meal I once made with only pears and cinnamon). Luckily, my parents were always supportive and very patient in these creative yet sometimes unappetizing endeavors, and ultimately gave me the space to explore food with full autonomy. Cooking became a ritual of comfort as I grew older and moved away from my childhood home, returning to familiar recipes to ground me in whatever country I called home at the time. And this soon became my most fluent love language and an active way in which I celebrated and honored my cultural legacy.

I grew up in a close-knit Japanese American community in Chicago. Being ethnically Japanese meant fermented and pickled products were a staple for nearly everything we made—cloudy miso soup, sweet soy sauce-glazed chicken wings, aromatic pickled cucumbers—be it at weekly Sunday night dinners with my grandparents or potluck meals at my Buddhist temple. But as we were also very American, my great-grandparents having immigrated to the USA at the end of the nineteenth century, we valued all of the convenience our home offered. Why would we make miso or soy sauce at home if we could easily buy everything, and was it worth the effort? While my life choices have clearly departed from this line of thought, I still subscribe to the idea that convenient options can be swapped in when necessary (and all my recipes in this book work with store-bought ferments and pickles).

These fermented flavors held deep meaning for my family and community. Umami, sourness, funk, the quintessential Japanese savory sweetness. For my grandparents and elders, who had a complicated history with the USA, these flavors were sources of comfort and a way in which to connect with our culture and honor our contribution to the patchwork quilt of America.

As my world opened up, going from college on the East Coast of the USA to working and living in Mumbai, New York, Hong Kong, and now London, I realized how universal the flavors unearthed through preservation are, not only in our collective memory but also in what they mean to us personally. The sourness of sauerkraut. A drizzle of soy sauce. The crunch of a dill pickle. These senses trigger memories of grandparents, of "weird" flavors we didn't appreciate as children but now crave as adults, of glass jars with cloudy liquid gathering dust, ingredients and techniques born through survival transporting you to those years of childhood wonder. Nostalgia.

This constant search for flavor in the places I've called home has allowed me to reframe my view of preservation through a global lens. Connecting the dots between diasporic traditions and the familiar pickles and ferments I grew up with brings me immense joy. But most importantly, this methodology is the foundation of how I approach food in my London home as a Japanese American, living life as a third-culture adult in a global kitchen.

Transforming food through preservation with a focus on low waste, locality, and seasonality has become incredibly trendy and could be perceived as a radical act, especially against today's backdrop of quick gratification and capitalistic food systems. The pandemic gave us time to reflect on who we are and what we eat, and we've emerged as a human race craving agency and control. Preserving at home takes us in the right direction.

I grew up in the 1990s when cultural norms pushed an antibacterial and sanitized agenda and this context can sometimes be the biggest mental hurdle. The pandemic undoubtedly exacerbated this fear of bacteria and viruses, but it was during that odd chapter of our lives that we simultaneously felt an urge to slow down. I saw friends who had never stepped into the kitchen before making sourdough, learning to live by the beat of their sourdough starter. Others started growing vegetables and herbs on their balconies, urban patches of land they could call their own.

In parallel, increased awareness of the gut microbiome and the health benefits of fermented products are accelerating at an exciting rate. Fermented foods play a large role in nurturing the gut, which in turn nurtures both our physical and mental well-being. However, we should remember and acknowledge that these traditions and food practices have always existed across the globe. A trend as old as time, learned through storytelling, intuition, muscle memory, taste, texture, and scent, and without a laboratory set-up.

This is not intended to be an exhaustive book but a guide and spark of creation. I have focused on some of the more accessible preservation techniques, which also reflect the popular preserved items available in today's supermarkets. With practice and increased confidence, you will make your own delicious creations, ones that honor traditions and also reflect your unique context. My recipes showcase these creations and show just what you can do with preserving. Long gone will be the days of having multiple jars of who-knows-what lurking in your fridge!

So let's learn together and dive head-first into the wonderful world of home preservation. Let this be the ripple that changes how you approach what nourishes both your body and soul. Let this be a point of departure in challenging how you eat and how you incorporate these building blocks of flavor into your everyday cooking. Enjoy the microbial ride and the inevitable rabbit holes as you preserve in your home kitchen. I promise you, this is only the beginning of the adventure.

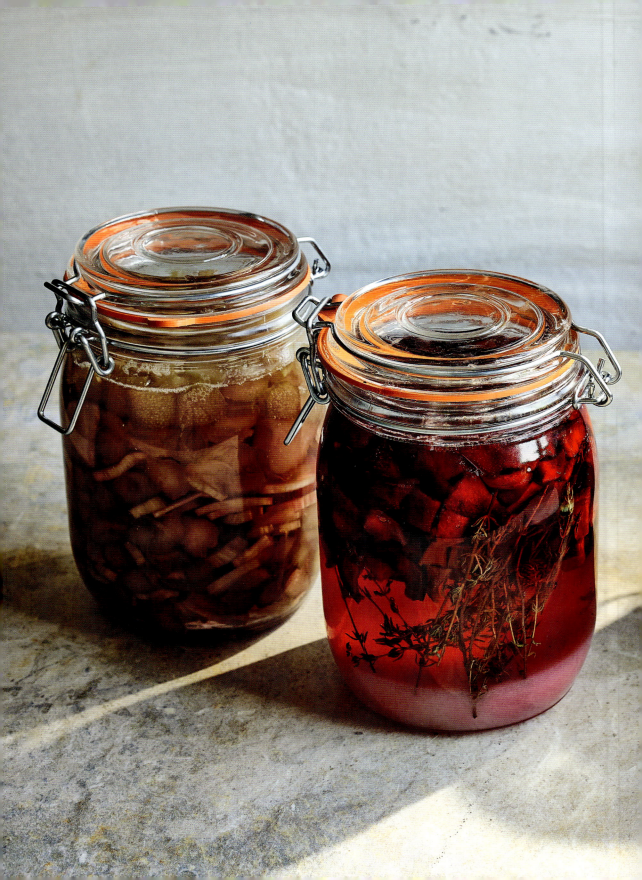

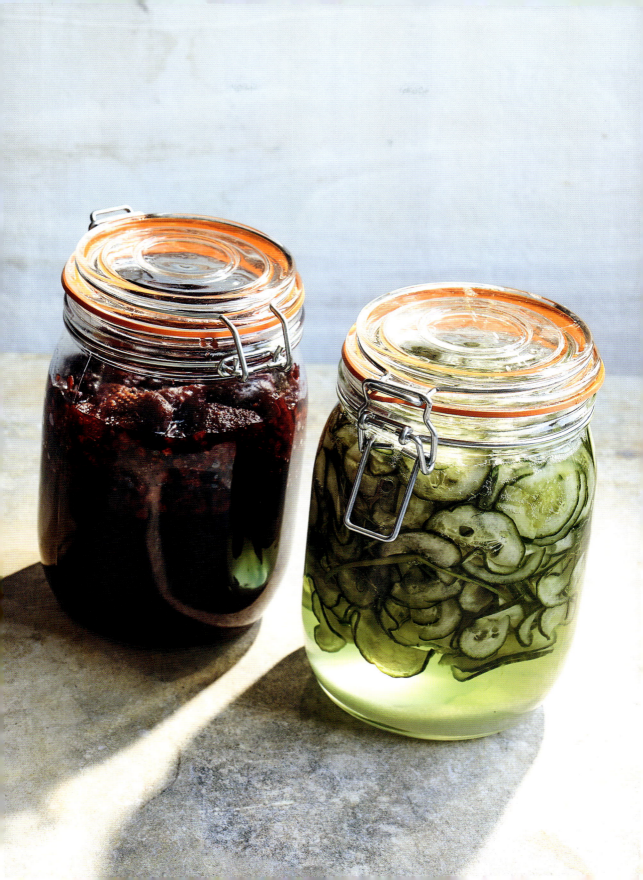

PRESERVATION 101

My approach to fermenting and pickling in a home kitchen is based on a few basic principles and is rooted in accessibility. I aim to reduce any obstacles, both in terms of new equipment or complicated and overly scientific methods, to show you just how easy it can be, with some preparation and adherence to best practices.

Everything I've learned and created has been within a home kitchen, with the attitude of a home cook. I do not have any fancy technical equipment and do not source the most expensive vegetables or artisanal salt. I use what I have, often following what's in season or checking for discounted produce, and I have learned to adjust my process based on my circumstances. This has, of course, led to numerous failings: unwanted yeast, scary-looking mold, and less than desirable flavor outcomes. But I've learned a lot from these mistakes, and this process of constant learning has yielded the best results, as well as a steadfast confidence in what I do.

An openness to failure is a necessary skill in the kitchen. View this book as a guide, to be adapted and built upon. Your unique environment will dictate the speed at which a sauerkraut ferments; how much salt you add is partly based on the time of the year and how you prepare your vegetables. While this potential variation in a cookbook may sound concerning, it's important to remember that we're working with living bacteria. Process can and should evolve based on the environment in which you're fermenting.

My mantras

Trust the process: Fermentation is a natural and transformative process. If the correct environment is created within your jar and the best practices below are followed, everything should be fine. Patience is key, as your individual environment (primarily referring to the temperature of your home kitchen) will impact the speed of fermentation. Remember that fermentation is sensory; below are some of the natural signs that fermentation is going as planned:

—You'll **see bubbles** and a build-up of carbon dioxide within the jar as the naturally occurring lactobacillus bacteria on the vegetables convert sugars into lactic acid, the necessary acidic environment for preservation and what gives fermented pickles their distinct flavor.

—You'll **hear hissing**, and see brine and vegetables rise to the top due to the creation of carbon dioxide. This is your cue to burp your jars (see page 17) and be on the lookout for any overspill of brine. Keeping your fermenting jars on a plate or shallow bowl will keep things tidy. You do not want to come home to a trail of brine leaking from your kitchen counter or splashed across your ceiling (both true stories).

—**Colors will change**: Vegetables' vibrancy may become muted and brine (when fermenting whole vegetables in a salty brine) will become cloudy.

Everything is fine below the brine: Most of the fermentation in this book is anaerobic, meaning that its magic works in the absence of oxygen. In the case of lactofermentation, as seen with sauerkraut and kimchi, it is important to minimize the vegetables' contact with oxygen. Using pressure (a pickle packer or wooden spoon) to compact the vegetables in your jar helps ensure there's a layer of brine between the vegetables and oxygen.

Anything sticking out of the brine, however small (a sliver of cabbage, a floating chile), will attract unwanted yeast or mold (more information on this on page 20 under "Cleanliness"). The best way to combat this is by using fermentation weights, which are commercially available, or a handful of DIY solutions which I outline below and on the next page. Note that there are some specific best practices for fermentation weights when making miso, which I'll dive into in that section (see pages 80–86).

—Use a small glass jar or food-safe cup which can fit into the mouth of the jar you're fermenting in. This is a particularly good option if you're using a swing-top jar as the pressure when you close it will force pressure onto whatever you're fermenting.

—Use a large cabbage leaf, slightly larger than the mouth of the jar—tuck the edges of the cabbage leaf down the sides of the jar and then give it a push to ensure the cabbage leaf barrier stays in place and the brine pools on top.

—Other options include a food-safe plastic bag filled with a salty brine, but the risk here is that it could leak into your ferment and impact the overall salt percentage.

In the absence of sufficient brine—which can easily happen as you start consuming your ferment and removing it from its packed environment—it's not uncommon for oxygen to make contact with the vegetables, which will lead to discoloration of your ferment (oxidation). This is not inherently bad and it is safe to eat unless covered in mold, but to avoid oxidation, keep the ferment packed under its brine and in the fridge for long-term storage.

You be the judge: Lactofermentation, as we will see in the next two sections, can happen quickly (sometimes in a matter of days). After the initial period of microbial activity, start tasting your pickles! If they need more tang, give them more time. If they're to your liking? Well, move them to the fridge to slow down the fermentation. Remember that as we are not pasteurizing our home ferments and pickles, they will continue to ferment, mature, and evolve—even in the fridge, although at a significantly slower rate.

Anyone who's made kimchi will know that its flavor and texture will change considerably throughout its fermentation life cycle: Fresher kimchi will be lighter in taste and often retain more of its crunch whereas older and more fermented kimchi will be funkier and therefore it is often used in cooking. While cooking will kill the good bacteria in the kimchi, it'll add heaps of flavor in ways a fresher kimchi would not.

Taste often, and remember to use a clean utensil every time!

Trust your gut: If something smells bad or is visibly covered in mold, throw it out (or better yet, compost it) and start again. The beauty of fermenting at home is that most of the ingredients are affordable, so it's not a massive loss as you start building your confidence with fermenting. Trust the process, keep everything below the brine, and use clean utensils and you should be in the clear. More information on page 20 on cleanliness when preserving at home.

Label everything: Always label your jars and projects—I like to use masking or painter's tape and permanent markers. Label with the name, date, and any relevant proportions or percentages used. The last thing you want is to lose track of this vital information, especially when you have many projects on the go at once. Alternatively, start a fermentation notebook to track all of this information, but in my experience, it's best (and more convenient) to label jars.

Equipment

Below are my suggested items for effective fermenting and pickling in your home kitchen, as well as best practices to optimize your success.

Digital kitchen scale: This is perhaps the most scientific element in how I approach preserving at home and is absolutely necessary for your home kitchen set-up. They are a great investment—with significant use going beyond the recipes in this book—and are affordable.

Fermentation requires a specific amount of salt to create the correct (and safe) environment for your food; it's calculated as a percentage of the weight of what you're fermenting. While I know our ancestors didn't have kitchen scales to measure exact grams of salt and I've heard stories of people (mainly elders) eyeballing the amount of salt needed with impressive accuracy, kitchen scales allow us to ferment with consistent results. So do yourself a favor and get a kitchen scale!

In the case of lactofermentation, most salt percentages range from 2–5%, so a kitchen scale is necessary to weigh the produce (and water, in the case of a wet brine—more information on page 32). You can then compute (with a handy calculator) the amount of salt needed.

For example, if you're making sauerkraut from 500g (1lb 2oz) of cabbage, you will need 10g (0.33oz) of salt if using 2% salt for the dry brine.

500g (1lb 2oz) x 0.02 = 10g (0.33oz) of salt

Containers: I'm a sucker for glass jars. They are inexpensive, reusable, and, as someone who appreciates the aesthetics of preservation, a perfect way to showcase your projects. Glass jars are also ideal since you can observe your ferment and make adjustments if needed. You can see what's happening below the brine or identify air pockets once it's jarred up—and when making miso, observe that glistening tamari.

There are many types of glass jars on the market and my favorite are flip-top glass jars: Both the jar and lid are glass and the flip-top mechanism allows for carbon dioxide to escape during the fermentation process.

That said, I ferment and pickle in all kinds of glass jars. Best practices vary depending on the type of jar being used:

—Traditional preservation jars with metal screw-top lids: Metal and acid isn't a good combination as it can lead to corrosion over long exposure. In my experience, this generally is not a problem in the

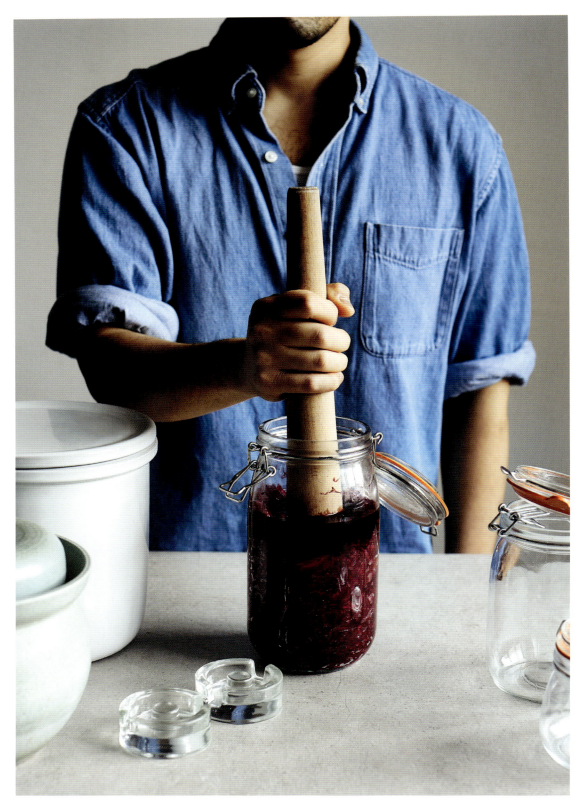

home setting, especially if you ensure that there is no existing rust on the lids. That said, many standard-size glass jars have food-safe reusable plastic alternatives for their lids. If using the metal screw-tops, don't screw the lids too tightly as this can lead to significant pressure build-up.

—Fermentation-specific glass jars: There are jars available that include air-locks, allowing carbon dioxide to escape but minimizing oxygen exposure and thereby removing the need to burp your jars. These are good entry-level jars if you're particularly nervous about yeast or mold. However, in my experience, they aren't necessary (and remember our ancestors didn't have access to them when fermenting). But who can put a price on that extra peace of mind?

—Old-school ceramic fermentation crocks: These have the added benefit that they have a water seal (which needs to be topped up as the water evaporates), creating an anaerobic environment by allowing carbon dioxide to escape and minimizing oxygen contact. But as someone who is relatively frugal and enjoys the aesthetics of preserving in glass jars, glass is my go-to for everything I create, be it a ferment, vinegar-based pickle, or miso.

I must remind you that most fermentation historically happened in an open vessel, which inevitably attracts unwanted mold and yeast. Regardless, when choosing your ideal jar—both in terms of type and size—always choose one according to what you're preserving: one that isn't too large (to minimize the amount of oxygen in the jar) but is also large enough to leave some headspace—ideally about 5cm (2in)—at the top of the jar. Carbon dioxide will push your pickles and brine up when the fermentation is particularly active (usually within the first week), which is why you need to keep your jar on a plate to catch any overflowing brine.

There's always a risk, particularly with kombucha and hot sauces in my experience, that the pressure can really build within the bottle. Any kombucha maker will tell you stories of popping bottles, which can be both dangerous and scary. While this has never happened to me while fermenting vegetables, the stories serve as reminders to burp our jars. Regardless of which type of jar you use, burp them regularly: This means slowly opening and closing the lid to let excess carbon dioxide escape.

Pickle packer: Visually similar to a wooden rolling pin (see photo opposite), these commercially available wooden tools help you pack your ferments tightly into your containers, allowing the brine to rise to the top and minimize oxygen exposure. Alternative options include a wooden spoon or even your bare hands, but I do recommend this tool for ease and efficiency.

Ingredients

The search for the best-quality cabbage or salt should not be a limiting factor when preserving at home. Use what you have access to and what you can afford. That said, as with most food, the quality of your ingredients will impact the quality of your end product.

For all recipes, rinse vegetables and fruits as you normally would with fresh water. Peeling vegetables is generally not required unless the recipe specifies otherwise; remember that the skin of vegetables and fruits contains a host of healthy bacteria needed for fermentation! Also, approach these methods through the lens of minimizing waste in your home kitchen. Preservation inherently tackles this, however, I challenge you to use as much of the vegetable or fruit as possible. For example, when making sauerkraut, I use as much of the cabbage core as possible in addition to the leaves. The key here is to ensure that it's prepared uniformly which allows the method in question to pickle or ferment at the same rate. I always feel a tremendous sense of accomplishment when my food waste from a project is at an absolute minimum.

In terms of salt, I generally stick with sea salt and avoid any salts that contain iodine and anti-caking agents as a best practice, as they can potentially inhibit fermentation.

Cleanliness

Cleanliness is key for success in preservation, particularly with fermentation, where unwanted bacteria can cause problems. As my focus is within a home setting and I do not sell my goods, I do not sterilize my jars in boiling water or in the oven; I simply wash them well using soap and water and let them air dry before using them. This is true for everything in this book.

A common concern among beginner fermenters is the fear of botulism, a bacteria-borne illness which many associate with home preservation. It's important to note that the environment for fermentation covered in this book is not hospitable to the bacteria that cause botulism; these particular bacteria usually live in low-acid and low-salt (as well as anaerobic) environments. There is no real risk if the best practices are followed. Botulism can be a concern for other forms of food preservation, such as canning, which is not a method covered in this book.

Contamination or yeast/mold growth are usually introduced to your ferment by unclean utensils and are most often seen as kahm yeast, a wild strain of yeast which forms a snow-like blanket on the surface of your ferment where oxygen meets the brine. Kahm yeast is harmless but is easily attracted by vegetables protruding from the brine (remember, everything is fine below the brine!). It is best to remove it as soon as possible as it can impact the flavor of your ferment and can attract mold if not dealt with quickly. You can do this simply by using a spoon or paper towel to remove it. It will not be possible to remove it entirely as once it's present in your ferment, it's "contaminated" with that wild yeast, but it can be kept at bay by moving the ferment to the fridge or keeping a watchful eye on the ferment as it continues developing. However, if it's moldy, it's time to start over.

Environment

As with most living things, our environment has a tremendous impact on the bacteria in pickles and ferments. A few top tips:

—Avoid direct sunlight: While it may be pretty to see your pickles illuminated with natural light, this can lead to temperature fluctuations and negatively impact your end product. A consistent environment is key, so I tend to leave my jars in cabinets or in dark corners of a room where they see only indirect light with the passing day's sun.

—Temperature: Based on where you live and at what point of the year you start a project, the salt content of your pickle can be adjusted to optimize the success rate. Many ferments across the globe historically were started during colder seasons, which meant a slower and more nuanced ferment. If you live in a warmer climate or start a project in the summer months, fermentation will generally be faster and more salt can be added at the start to ensure safety. For lactofermentation, I generally ferment sauerkrauts at 2% salt and whole vegetables/hot sauces in a wet brine at 3–4%. Feel free to increase this slightly based on where you live but I'd generally stay within the 2–5% range for lactofermentation.

And lastly, focus on the basics: Learn what works best for you, and then, once you feel confident in your foundation, let that spark your discovery of new flavors.

INTRODUCTION

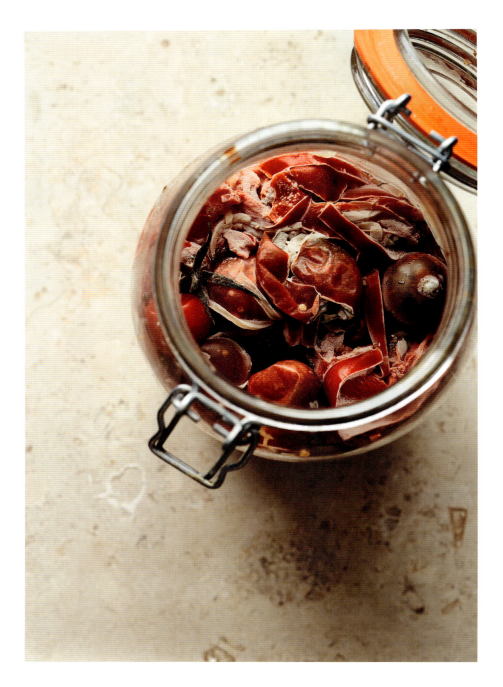

Above: The early stages of kahm yeast blooms due to the fermenting vegetables being above the brine. Opposite: Here I've used a piece of parchment paper to ensure that my Zero-Waste Green Paste (page 40) stays "fine below the brine."

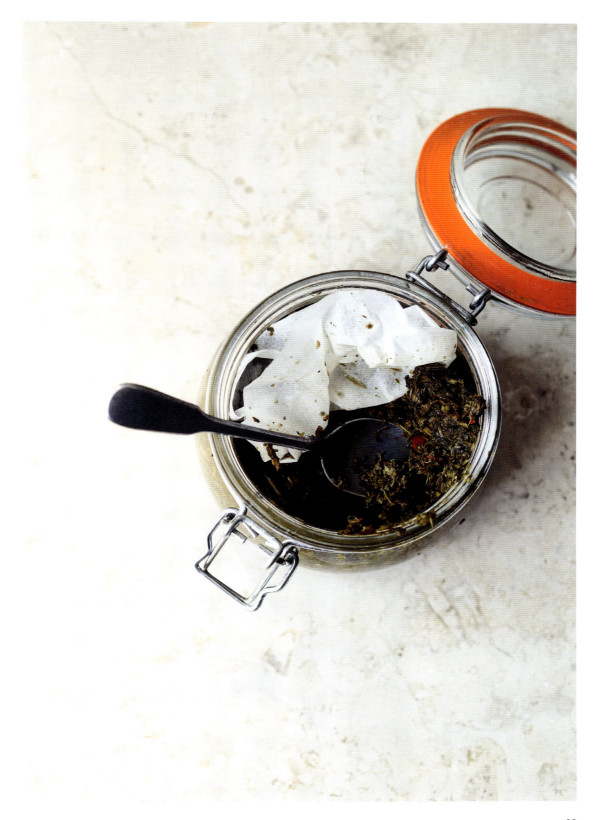

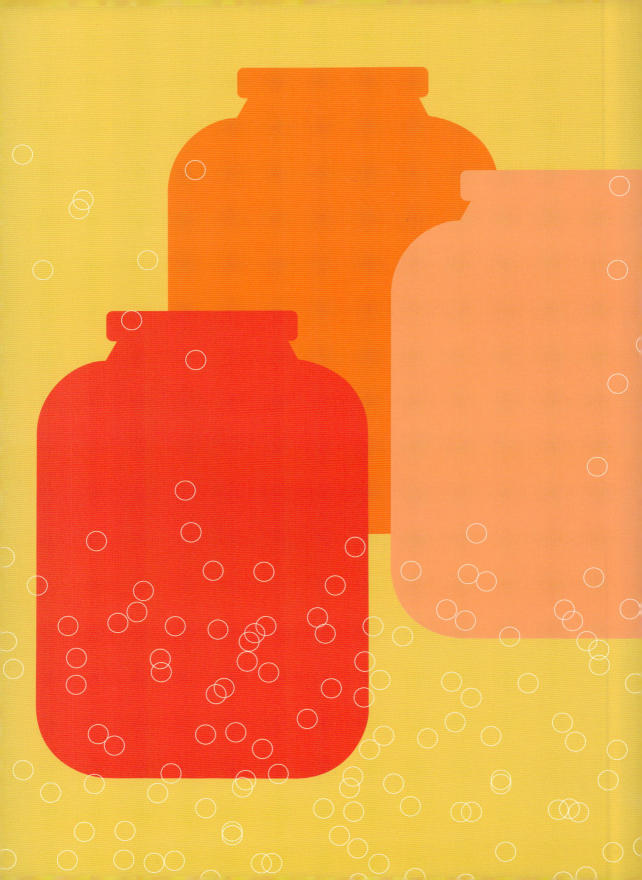

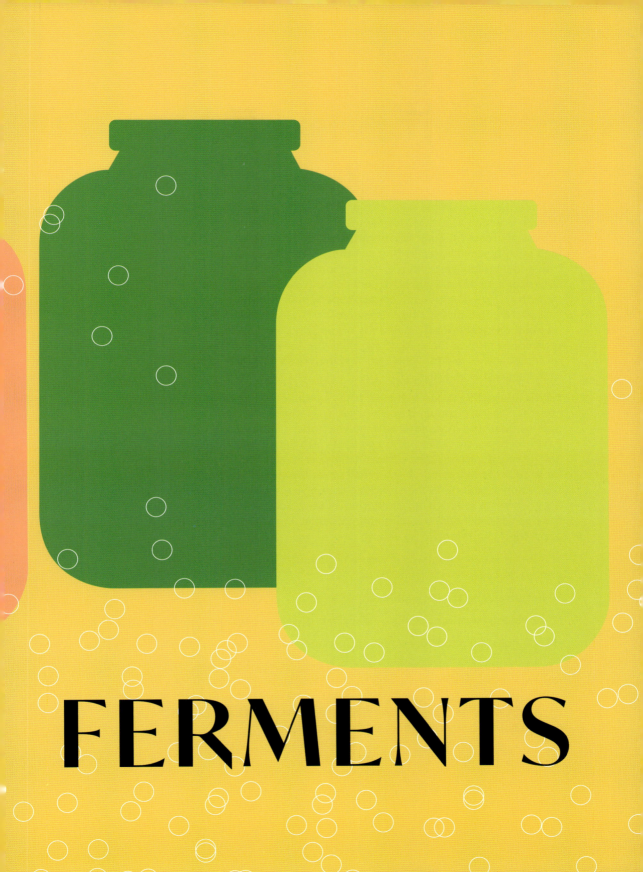

LACTO-FERMENTATION

Lactofermentation is the microbial process behind sauerkraut and kimchi, in which a salty environment accomplishes two important drivers of preservation. It kills harmful bacteria that cannot survive high salinity while also allowing lactobacillus bacteria—present on fruit and vegetables—to thrive, consuming the naturally present sugars and creating lactic acid. Lactic acid (which has nothing to do with dairy, a common misconception) both preserves and gives these fermented pickles their unique taste. There are two main techniques, descriptively called dry brining and wet brining. These techniques refer to the method by which the salty brine is created for lactobacillus to work its magic. The method is usually a reflection of the vegetable you're using.

Dry brining: This is generally used for vegetables with high water content. They are chopped or shredded to increase surface area. Salt is added and massaged into the vegetables with force to create a natural brine. By cutting the vegetables into thin or small pieces and increasing their surface area, you maximize the opportunity for brine to be extracted as you break down the cellular walls. The best-known example is the shredded cabbage used for sauerkraut. It's possible to create a dry brine from larger pieces of vegetables, but this will most definitely require more time and could increase the opportunity for things to go wrong.

I often get asked what to do if there's not enough liquid from the dry brining process. This is normally due to:

(1) not shredding the vegetables thinly enough

(2) not using fresh vegetables—older ones have lower water content

(3) not massaging the vegetables with enough force

If you're struggling, keep at it or, after a substantial massage, let the vegetables continue to salt at room temperature before packing them into your container of choice. Do not add a salty brine to top up the dry brine as this will bring the salt content out of balance and could have a detrimental effect on the end product.

Wet brining: This is generally used for vegetables with lower water content or vegetables left in larger pieces. A salty brine is added to vegetables when brine can not be extracted by the dry brining process. Use this method to ferment whole chiles and aromatics for a hot sauce to be blended post-fermentation, larger vegetable pieces for a zingy crudité, or whole dill cucumbers—all recipes incoming!

Once your jar is filled with vegetables in a salty brine and you ensure everything is below the brine, the anaerobic fermentation process will begin and within a few days you'll start to witness the magic: bubbles, hissing, the need to burp the jar, the once-vibrant colors of your vegetables slightly muted, once-clear brine now cloudy. When the ferment settles down, usually after a minimum of a week, taste your ferment and move it to the fridge (decanting it into smaller jars if easier) when you're pleased with its flavor. It's important that you continue to tamp the vegetables down and keep everything below the brine; if you don't, you risk oxidation (which will generally look like slight discoloration) or potential yeast or mold.

I tend to lactoferment at room temperature for a minimum of a week, but have some ferments going on for months: batches of sauerkraut, whole chiles for hot sauce, green tomatoes from the garden, as well as quartered cabbages, all fermenting at room temperature. A treasure trove of flavorful building blocks, ready to be tasted and explored.

I'll dive into these further in my basic recipes for both methods, followed by some of my favorite creative twists that have become mainstays in my home kitchen. And always remember to keep your brine when wet brining—it can kickstart a new ferment, is a massive source of flavor, and can be used endlessly in the kitchen. Always taste it to determine how it can benefit a dish: thrown into sauces, dressings, brines for meat ahead of a barbecue, or even in a cheeky cocktail.

DRY BRINING 101

This method is for vegetables with high water content (such as cabbage), or vegetables processed in a way (finely shredded or thinly cut) that optimizes surface area and allows brine to be created from the vegetables themselves.

- Thinly slice or uniformly shred the vegetables; this can be done by hand or carefully with a mandoline.

- Put a large bowl onto a digital kitchen scale and zero it out. Weigh the prepared vegetables and calculate 2% of the total weight. For example, if the total weight of cabbage is 1kg (2.25lbs), you will need 20g (0.75oz) of salt; 2% salt is the standard proportion I use for dry brining.
  If you want to add dry spices, no need to factor them in as their nominal weight won't impact the proportions.

- In the same large bowl, sprinkle the salt onto the prepared vegetables and give them a strong massage with your hands. The force from the massage will break down the cell walls of the vegetables and extract water, which will combine with the salt to create the brine needed for safe preservation. This may take some time—depending on the freshness of your vegetables and how thinly you cut them—and can take up to 5–10 minutes of continuous pressure.

- Decant the massaged vegetables and brine into your jar of choice, ensuring there's adequate headspace—ideally about 5cm (2in) – at the top of the jar.

- Pack it all in with a wooden spoon or wooden pickle packer to ensure there are no pockets of air among the vegetables. There should be a layer of brine at the top of your packed vegetables. Do your best to push all of the vegetables below the brine. If there is not enough brine at this stage—i.e., a clear layer of brine between the vegetables and air—return the vegetables to the bowl and continue with the massage to allow the salt to extract more brine.

- Use a food-safe fermentation weight (see pages 15–16) to hold down any floating bits of vegetables. Remember that anything above the brine could attract unwanted yeast or mold.

—Cover the jar with its lid—slightly ajar if using a screw-top jar—and leave it at room temperature out of direct sunlight for up to 2 weeks. Keep the jar on a plate or shallow bowl to catch any overspill of brine. The main fermentation process will start in a few days. Over the next 2 weeks, you'll notice the signs of fermentation. As bacteria consume sugars and create acid in the salty environment, carbon dioxide is created: You'll see bubbles and will need to burp your jar (see page 19).

—After the initial 5 days of fermentation (or less in a warm kitchen), start tasting (and smelling). If you're happy with the taste, move the jar to the fridge for long-term storage. For more sourness, continue to ferment at room temperature. If you're maintaining the best practices, you can keep it indefinitely in the fridge or at room temperature; however, the texture and flavors will change, so move it to the fridge when you're satisfied.

If anything doesn't look as you expected, return to my Preservation 101 section (pages 14–21) which covers the process in more detail.

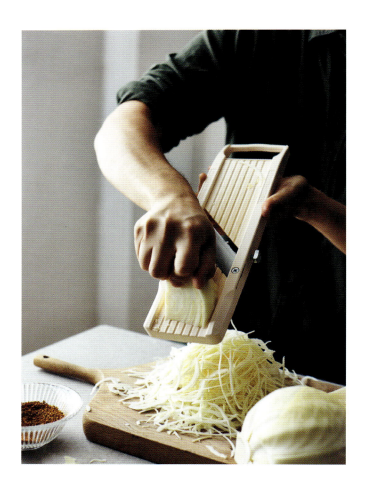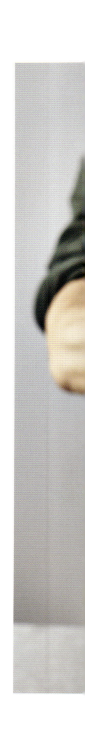

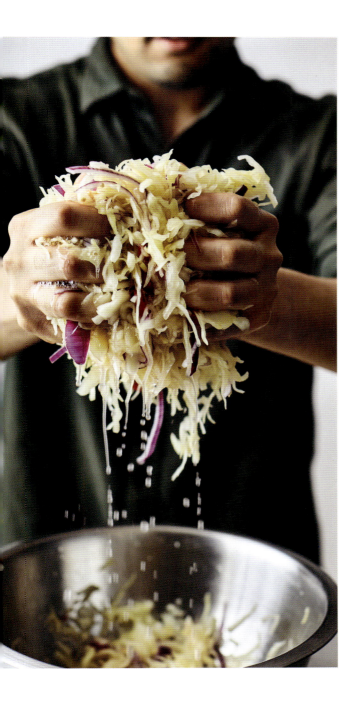
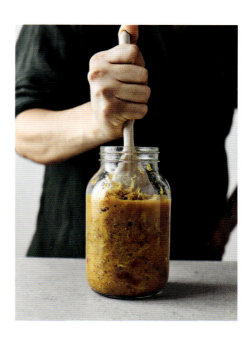

WET BRINING 101

This method is for vegetables with lower water content or vegetables that are left whole or in larger pieces, such as chiles, carrots, whole cucumbers, and tomatoes. Note that the amount of salt added depends on the total weight of everything inside the jar—vegetables AND water—therefore the recipe will change based on container size; however, the percentages and proportions stay the same.

—Prepare your vegetables—these may be left whole or cut into smaller pieces to fit into a jar.

—Find a jar that will hold your vegetables. Put this onto your digital kitchen scale and zero it out. Fill up the jar with whatever you're fermenting (fresh vegetables, herbs, and dried spices) and add water until everything is submerged. Take a note of that total weight. It is usually best to add a bit more water as this will help to keep what you're fermenting below the brine; however, leave some headspace—ideally about 5cm (2in)—to allow for microbial activity.

—Calculate 3–4% of the total weight of everything in the jar. For example, if the total weight is 2kg (4lbs 6oz) you will need 60–80g (2–3oz) of salt. Add the salt, close the jar, and shake to dissolve.

—Use a food-safe fermentation weight (see pages 15–16) to hold down any floating bits of vegetables. Remember that anything above the brine could attract unwanted yeast or mold.

—Cover the jar with its lid—slightly ajar if using a screw-top jar—and leave it at room temperature out of direct sunlight for a minimum of 5 days and up to several weeks. Keep the jar on a plate or shallow bowl to catch any overspill of brine. The main fermentation process will start pretty immediately. During this time, you'll notice the signs of fermentation. As bacteria consume sugars and create acid in the salty environment, carbon dioxide is created: You'll see bubbles and will need to burp your jar (see page 19).

—After the initial 5 days of fermentation (or less in a warm kitchen), start tasting (and smelling). If you're happy with the taste, move the jar to the fridge for long-term storage. For more sourness, continue to ferment at room temperature. If you're maintaining the best practices, you can keep it indefinitely in the fridge or at room temperature; however, the texture and flavors will change, so move it to the fridge when you're satisfied.

If it doesn't look right, return to Preservation 101 (pages 14–21).

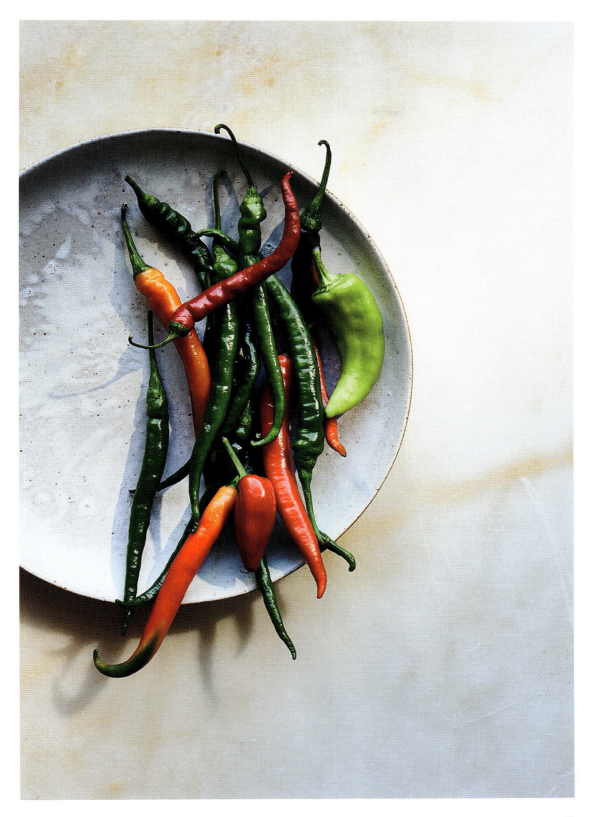

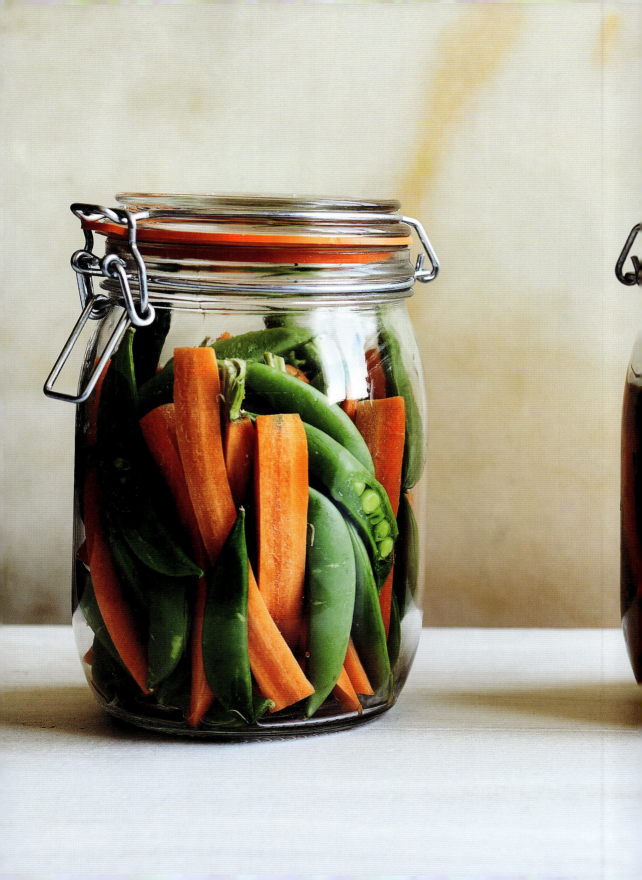

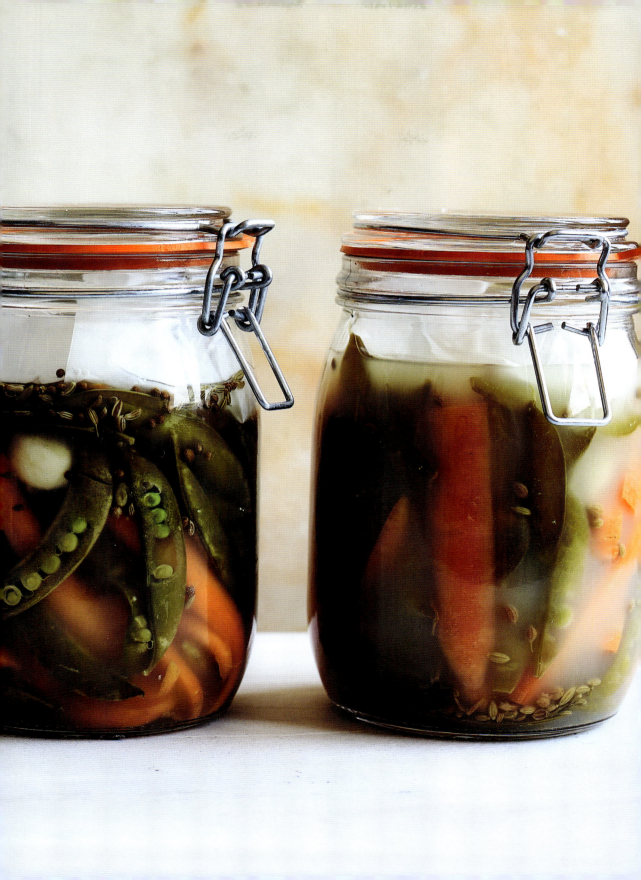

GARAM MASALA SAUERKRAUT

This is my favorite variety of sauerkraut and was the first fun flavor profile I explored after I was confident with the basics. If you want to make this recipe even easier, swap the individual spices for a ready-made curry or garam masala blend; however, dry roasting the spices first and then freshly grinding them will release the natural oils and impart much more flavor, so it's worth this additional step. This sauerkraut is incredible in a grilled cheese, the spices adding a lovely warmth to the melted cheese; mix it into a chicken salad or eat it alongside your next South Asian feast. *See step-by-step images on pages 30–31.*

PREP TIME: 30–45 MINUTES | FERMENTATION TIME: 2–5 WEEKS

Makes one 1-liter (1-quart) jar

- 800g (1.75lbs) white cabbage
- 1 small red onion about 100g/3.5oz, peeled and thinly sliced
- 2 mild red chiles about 30g (1oz), deseeded and thinly sliced
- measured salt: 2% of the total weight of above ingredients

FOR THE SPICE MIX

- 1 tbsp coriander seeds
- 1 tbsp cumin seeds
- 2 tsp brown mustard seeds
- 1 tsp black peppercorns
- 1 tsp fennel seeds
- 2 green cardamom pods, crushed and seeds extracted
- ¼ tsp red pepper flakes
- 1 tsp ground turmeric

Halve the cabbage. Shred it finely using a sharp knife or a mandoline. Place the shredded cabbage in a bowl with the red onion and chiles and calculate 2% of the total weight. This is the amount of salt you need.

Add the salt to the vegetables and massage for 5–10 minutes, using a fair amount of pressure to optimize the creation of brine. If you do not see much brine, continue massaging the cabbage and a pool of brine should appear.

Put all of the ingredients for the spice mix except the turmeric into a dry pan over a medium heat for 1–2 minutes until aromatic and the mustard seeds start to pop. Tip into a spice blender and blitz only a few times until it's a coarse mixture; you can also do this using a mortar and pestle.

Add the spice mixture and the turmeric to the vegetables and mix thoroughly.

Decant into a jar and pack it down to ensure there are no air pockets, allowing the brine to gather on top of the vegetables. Use a food-safe fermentation weight to ensure everything is below the brine.

Cover the jar and leave it at room temperature and out of direct sunlight for 2–5 weeks. After 2 weeks, start tasting. When you're pleased with the flavor, move it to the fridge where it will keep indefinitely.

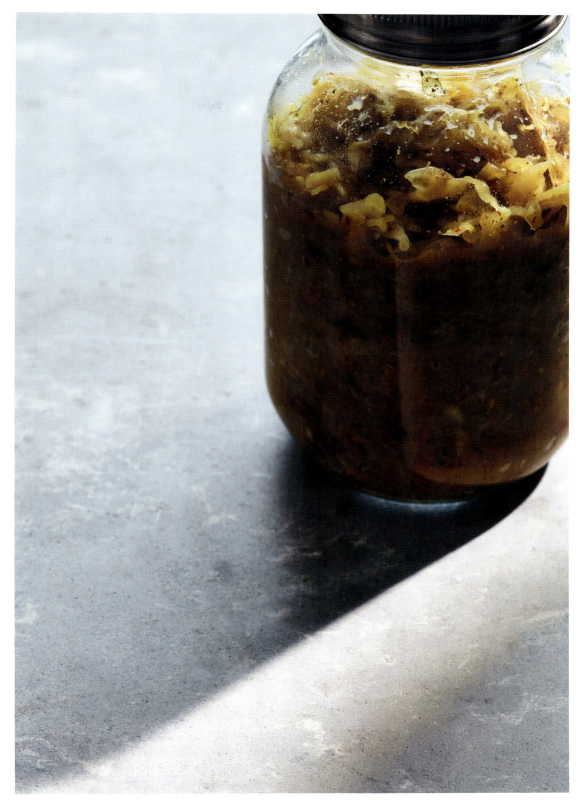

FERMENTED CRUDITÉS

This can be made with any of your favorite crudité vegetables and you can adjust the spices to your own preference: I've gone with carrots and sugar snap peas, but use what you have or what looks good at the store! Some of my other favorite vegetables include green beans, broccolini, asparagus, or baby red peppers. The most important thing is the salt brine—a percentage of the weight of everything that's inside the jar—and this means you can get creative with what goes in! Make sure all the vegetables are cut to a similar size so they ferment at the same pace.

Fermented crudités are delicious on a snack platter, alongside fresh vegetables to show the difference in flavor, and are a great way to use up odds and ends if you're heading out for the weekend and need to rescue vegetables in your fridge! *See the stages of fermenting on pages 34–35.*

PREP TIME: 15 MINUTES | FERMENTATION TIME: 5–7 DAYS

Makes one 2-liter (2-quart) jar

- 800g (1.75lbs) carrots, peeled and cut into batons
- 240g (8.5oz) sugar snap peas, left whole
- 2 garlic cloves, peeled
- 1 tbsp coriander seeds
- 1 tbsp fennel seeds
- measured salt: 3.5% of the total weight of above ingredients and water

Find a jar that will hold all your vegetables. Put this onto your kitchen scale and zero it out. Fill the jar with the vegetables, garlic, spices, and water and take a note of the total weight. (It is usually best to add a bit more water as this will help to keep what you're fermenting below the brine.)

Calculate 3.5% of the total weight. This is the amount of salt you will need. Add the salt to the jar, close the jar, and shake to dissolve.

Use a food-safe fermentation weight to hold down any floating vegetable bits below the brine.

Ferment at room temperature for 5–7 days. When you notice the signs of fermentation (see page 32), taste the vegetables: They should be tangy and effervescent. Move them to the fridge for long-term storage—they should keep for several months as long as they stay below the brine. In my opinion, these are best eaten when they're lightly fermented, both in terms of flavor and texture.

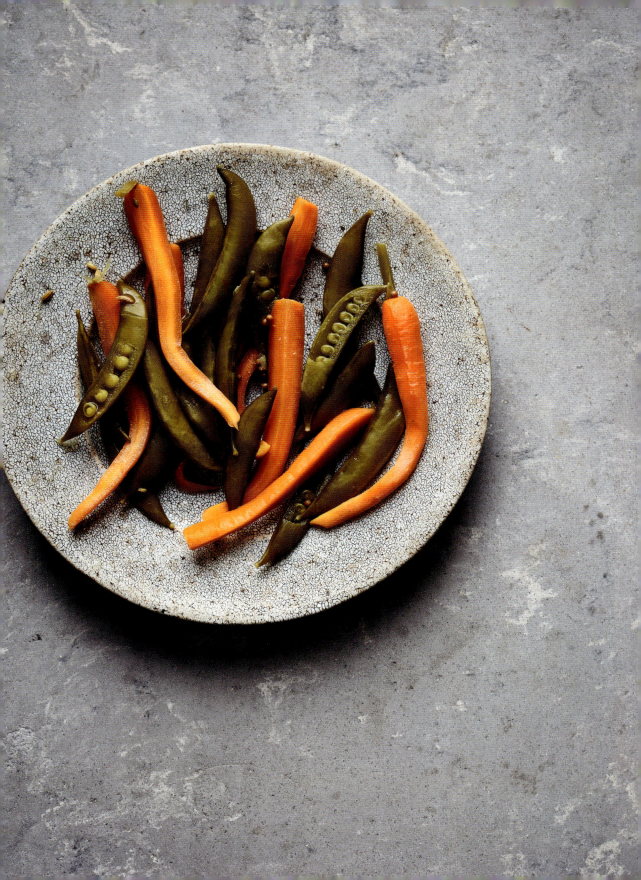

ZERO-WASTE GREEN PASTE

One of my toxic traits is that I'll buy fresh herbs in bulk with grand ambitions; fast forward a week and they're languishing in the back of my fridge, past their prime and objectively sad. Can anyone else relate to that?

Fermentation is the answer to this problem. This recipe is scalable and you can make it with almost any combination of herbs and aromatics; the ones opposite are those I normally have in my fridge needing salvation. Have dill and green onion or parsley and fresh turmeric? Then use those (or whatever else needs a home) but remember that the flavors you ferment will impact the final profile of the green paste. I find the ingredients opposite are "universal" enough to be applied to many different cuisines: added to marinades for barbecued meat, pulsed with chickpeas to make hummus for a Mediterranean feast, or thrown into stir-fries and curries for an instant punch of flavor (as I've done with my Plant-Based Zero-Waste Green Curry on page 202).

As this is a paste, you may immediately struggle with the "everything is fine below the brine" mantra. Fermentation weights won't work too well (in my experience) so I generally cover the surface of the paste with a piece of parchment paper or plastic wrap to minimize exposure to oxygen. It can also attract kahm yeast (harmless but not ideal) and may oxidize slightly at the top. This is common when fermenting pastes, such as chile pastes, where there isn't an obvious layer of brine keeping the ferment anaerobic (see page 28). It is all safe to eat, but move it to the fridge after the initial fermentation period to slow down the process. Also, after each use, flatten the top of the paste with a clean utensil and cover with parchment paper or plastic wrap.

The photo for this recipe is on page 23.

PREP TIME: 10 MINUTES | FERMENTATION TIME: 7–10 DAYS

Makes one 500-ml (1-pint) jar

- 70g (2.5oz) fresh cilantro (leaves and stems), roughly chopped
- 70g (2.5oz) fresh mint (leaves and stems), roughly chopped
- 70g (2.5oz) fresh basil (leaves and stems), roughly chopped
- 35g (1.25oz) garlic cloves, peeled and roughly chopped
- 35g (1.25oz) fresh ginger, roughly chopped
- 110g (4oz) mixed chiles (deseeded if you want to reduce the heat level)
- measured salt: 4% of the total weight of above ingredients

SPECIAL EQUIPMENT: food processor

Find a jar that will hold all of the ingredients (apart from the salt). Put this onto your kitchen scale and zero it out. Fill the jar with the herbs, aromatics, and chiles and take a note of the total weight. Calculate 4% of the total weight. This is the amount of salt you will need.

Put all of the ingredients, including the salt, into a food processor and blitz until you have a coarse paste. (Depending on the size and weight of your food processor, you could put it directly on the kitchen scale.)

Using a spatula, decant the paste into the jar. Minimize any air pockets by gently tapping the jar against a kitchen towel-covered counter. Do your best here, but as the paste ferments, additional brine will be pulled from the paste, which should fill any air pockets. Cover the surface of the paste with a piece of parchment paper or plastic wrap.

Ferment at room temperature for 7–10 days. When you notice the signs of fermentation (see page 29), taste the paste; when you're happy with the flavor, move it to the fridge for long-term storage. Remember that this is a spice paste so will be strong in flavor and salty! It will keep indefinitely in the fridge, but is best consumed within a few months.

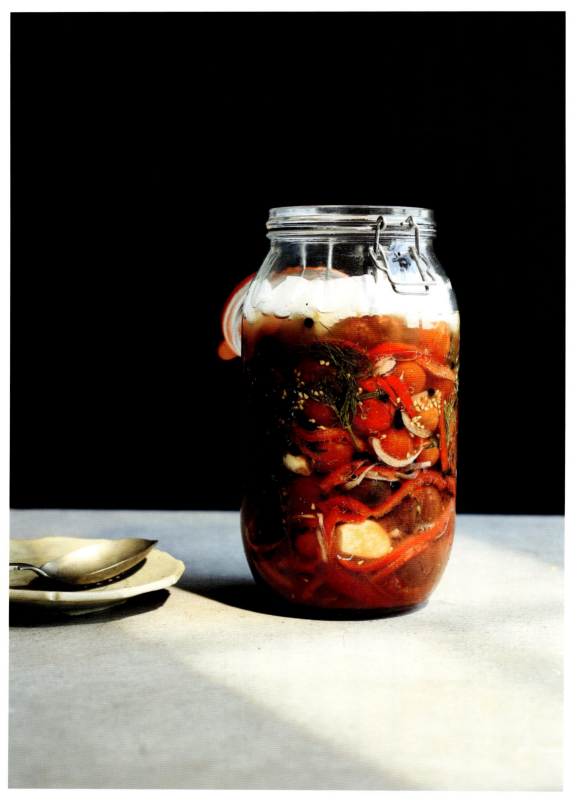

GAZPACHO CHERRY TOMATOES

Lactofermented cherry tomatoes are some of the best (and easiest) ferments you can make. There's something very special about biting into a fermented tomato: a burst of sweet and sour tang with a slight sparkly effervescence that just sings summer.

This ferment follows the wet brining process outlined on page 32. Here, I've leaned into the flavors of gazpacho, so I've added red pepper, red onion, chile, black peppercorns, and fresh dill. You can change up the ingredients or spices but remember to calculate the salt percentage based on the total weight of the ingredients and water.

These pickles and brine are the star of my Fermented Gazpacho (see page 162) and are particularly delicious in my Tomatini cocktail (see page 260). Keep any surplus brine for tomato sauces, a Bloody Mary, or dressings for summer salads.

PREP TIME: 20 MINUTES | FERMENTATION TIME: 5–7 DAYS

Makes one 1.5-liter (1.5-quart) jar

- **450g (1lb) cherry tomatoes, left whole**
- **5 garlic cloves, peeled**
- **1 red pepper (about 200g/7oz), deseeded and thinly sliced**
- **1 small red onion (about 100g/3.5oz), peeled, cut in half, and thinly sliced**
- **1 mild chile (10g/0.33oz), deseeded and roughly chopped**
- **2 tsp black peppercorns**
- **3–4 sprigs of fresh dill**
- **measured salt: 3.5% of the total weight of above ingredients and water**

Find a jar that will hold all of the ingredients (apart from the salt). Put this onto your kitchen scale and zero it out. Fill the jar with the vegetables, spices, herbs, and water and take a note of the total weight. (It is usually best to add a bit more water as this will help to keep what you're fermenting below the brine.) Calculate 3.5% of the total weight. This is the amount of salt you will need. Add the salt to the jar, close the jar, and shake to dissolve.

Use a food-safe fermentation weight to hold down any floating vegetable pieces. Remember that anything above the brine could attract unwanted yeast or mold.

Ferment at room temperature for 5–7 days. When you notice the signs of fermentation (see page 32), taste the tomatoes: They should be tangy and effervescent. Move them to the fridge for long-term storage—they should keep for several months as long as they stay below the brine. In my opinion, these are best eaten when they're lightly fermented, both in terms of flavor and texture.

SOUR DILL PICKLES

Most widely available cucumber pickles are vinegar based, which are delicious, but fermented cucumber pickles are superior in my humble opinion—not just in flavor, but also as a lesson in how fermentation affects sourness and texture. Ferment them for 3–4 days for "half sours" or double that time after which they're considered "full sours." I love the crunch at around the 10-day mark. As they ferment, the texture may get soft (even with the addition of bay leaves—dried or fresh—which contain tannins and help maintain the crunch) so you be the judge!

Feel free to change up the spices and herbs, but the one non-negotiable is the type of cucumber. Large water-dense cucumbers will not work; they'll inevitably go off and not ferment properly. Always use pickling cucumbers or other small varieties.

Slice these pickles and eat them on a burger or as a tangy vegetable in a salad such as my Curried Pickle Smashed Potato Salad (see page 185).

PREP TIME: 15 MINUTES | FERMENTATION TIME: 3–4 DAYS (half sour), 6+ DAYS (full sour)

Makes one 1.5-liter (1.5-quart) jar

- Approximately 600g (1lb 5oz) small pickling cucumbers (as many as can fit in the jar)
- 1 tsp yellow mustard seeds
- 1 tsp coriander seeds
- 1 tsp fennel seeds
- 1 tsp allspice, ground or whole berries
- ½ tsp ground turmeric
- ¼ tsp red pepper flakes
- 3–4 whole cloves
- 1 star anise
- 2 bay leaves, fresh or dried
- 4–5 sprigs of fresh dill (about 25g/1oz)
- 3–4 garlic cloves, peeled and left whole
- 2–3 chiles, left whole
- measured salt: 3.5% of the total weight of above ingredients and water

First prepare your cucumbers by trimming off both ends; the blossom end of the cucumber contains an enzyme which will soften the cucumber as it ferments, so doing this will help retain its crunch.

Find a jar that will hold your vegetables. Put the jar onto your kitchen scale and zero it out. Add the dried spices, bay leaves, fresh dill, garlic, and chiles. Then layer in the cucumbers.

Fill the jar with water. Note the total weight of everything in the jar. Calculate 3.5% of the total weight. This is the amount of salt you will need. Add the salt to the jar, close the jar, and shake to dissolve.

Use a food-safe fermentation weight to hold down any floating vegetable bits below the brine.

Ferment at room temperature. Taste at the two intervals for half and full sour (see above) to determine what you like. I prefer the longer fermented, very sour pickles. When you're happy with the taste and tang, move them to the fridge for long-term storage. (I think they're best when cold and straight from the fridge, which helps retain the crunch!) They should keep for several months as long as they stay below the brine.

EVERYDAY HOT SAUCE

This is another solution for chiles and aromatics that can get neglected in my fridge. It's a fairly standard hot sauce in terms of ingredients (chiles, garlic, and onion) and, as a result, can be used for a host of dishes. The fermentation process brings a wonderful tang and complexity of flavor, with a welcoming (and lingering) heat which makes it very versatile.

Keep the ingredients whole to be added to salsas or slow braises. Blitz to a chunky consistency to use as a traditional chile paste or as part of a marinade, bringing heat and flavor. Or purée to a sauce-like consistency, as shown below.

PREP TIME: 15 MINUTES | FERMENTATION TIME: 2 WEEKS minimum

Makes one 1-liter (1-quart) jar

- 200g (7oz) mixed chiles, stems removed, left whole if small or cut in half if larger
- 15–20g (0.5–0.75oz) hot chiles, such as bird's eye or Scotch bonnet, stems removed, left whole if smaller varieties
- 1 head of garlic, cloves peeled and crushed
- 1 small onion, peeled and roughly chopped
- 1 tsp black peppercorns
- ½ tsp red pepper flakes
- measured salt: 3.5% of the total weight of above ingredients and water
- Apple cider vinegar (optional)

SPECIAL EQUIPMENT: food processor or blender

Find a jar that will hold your chiles, garlic, and onion. Put this onto your kitchen scale and zero it out. Fill the jar with the vegetables, spices, and water and take a note of that total weight. (It is usually best to add a bit more water, as this will help to keep what you're fermenting below the brine).

Calculate 3.5% of the total weight. This is the amount of salt you will need. Add the salt to the jar, cover the jar, and shake well.

Use a food-safe fermentation weight to hold down any floating vegetable bits below the brine.

Ferment at room temperature for a minimum of 2 weeks. You can ferment this for much longer (I have fermented some pre-blended hot sauces for over a year at room temperature).

When you're ready to make the hot sauce, strain the ingredients (reserving the leftover brine). Put the ingredients into a food processor or blender and blitz to your desired consistency. At this point, your hot sauce is done.

If you want to loosen it, add some of the reserved brine or some apple cider vinegar, if using. Vinegar is often used for fermented hot sauces as it increases the acidity, making the sauce more shelf stable. That said, I'd suggest keeping blended hot sauces in the fridge as they can easily attract unwanted yeast.

LACTO FERMENTATION

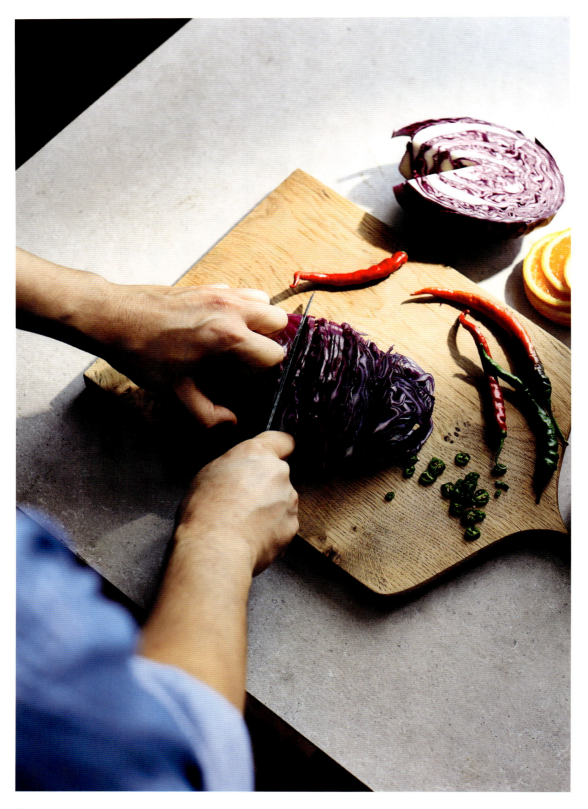

CHILE, ORANGE & CORIANDER SAUERKRAUT

As someone who makes a lot of sauerkraut, this is one variety that I return to quite often. It's really bright—not just in color from the ruby-red cabbage, but also in flavor from the orange playing off coriander's citrus notes. It really shines on a pickle platter and, with its fairly universal flavors, can be eaten alongside most cuisines. It's also particularly beautiful when baked into my Sauercaccia (see page 156).

PREP TIME: 15 MINUTES | FERMENTATION TIME: 2–5 WEEKS

Makes one 1-liter (1-quart) jar

1kg (2.25lbs) red cabbage

1 orange (peel included), thinly sliced

2 mild chiles, thinly sliced (deseeded if you want to reduce the heat level)

measured salt: 2% of the total weight of above ingredients

1 tbsp coriander seeds

Halve the cabbage. Shred it finely using a sharp knife or a mandoline—I like to use as much of the cabbage as possible. Place the shredded cabbage in a bowl with the orange and chiles and calculate 2% of the total weight. This is the amount of salt you will need.

Remove the orange slices and set aside. Add the salt to the sliced cabbage and chiles and massage for 5–10 minutes, using a fair amount of pressure to optimize the creation of brine. If you do not see much brine, continue massaging the cabbage and a pool of brine should appear. Add the sliced orange and coriander seeds and mix it all together.

Decant into a jar and pack it down to ensure there are no air pockets in your sauerkraut, allowing the brine to gather on top of the mixture. Use a food-safe fermentation weight to ensure everything is below the brine.

Cover the jar and leave it at room temperature and out of direct sunlight to ferment for 2–5 weeks. After 2 weeks, start tasting. When you're pleased with the flavor, move it to the fridge where it will keep indefinitely.

PINEAPPLE & SCOTCH BONNET HOT SAUCE

There are certain rituals that signal the start of a good weekend and one of those is a visit to my local market in Brixton, South London. Known for its West African and Caribbean communities, the market is a great place to find ingredients such as Scotch bonnets. This chile's fruity heat was new to me, but I immediately fell in love with it in my home cooking. When fermenting a hot sauce in a wet brine, I often find that the heat mellows but the flavors feel more pronounced, which is why I like to keep the ingredients quite straightforward. The garlic adds an aromatic note to the hot sauce, and the heat is balanced by the sweet pineapple. Spicy, summery, and an excellent addition to your hot sauce collection. Also delicious with grilled meats and marinades.

PREP TIME: 15 MINUTES | FERMENTATION TIME: 2 WEEKS minimum

Makes one 1–1.5-liter (1–1.5-quart) jar

- 500g (1lb 2oz) fresh pineapple, peeled and cut into large chunks (prepared weight)
- 70g (2.5oz) mixed chiles, stems removed, left whole
- 30g (1oz) Scotch bonnet chiles
- 20g (0.75oz) garlic (3–4 cloves), peeled and left whole
- ½ onion (about 70g/2.5oz), peeled and roughly chopped
- measured salt: 3.5% of the total weight of above ingredients and water
- Apple cider vinegar (optional)

SPECIAL EQUIPMENT: food processor or blender

Find a jar that will hold all of the ingredients (apart from the salt). Put this onto your kitchen scale and zero it out. Fill the jar with the pineapple, chiles, aromatics, and water and take a note of that total weight. (It is usually best to add a bit more water as this will help to keep what you're fermenting below the brine.)

Calculate 3.5% of the total weight. This is the amount of salt you will need. Add the salt to the jar, close the jar, and shake to dissolve.

Use a food-safe fermentation weight to hold down any floating vegetable bits below the brine.

Ferment at room temperature for a minimum of 2 weeks. You can ferment this for much longer (I have fermented some pre-blended hot sauces for over a year at room temperature).

When you're ready to make the hot sauce, strain the ingredients (reserving the leftover brine). Put the ingredients into a food processor or blender and blitz to your desired consistency. At this point, your hot sauce is done.

If you want to loosen it, you can add some of the reserved brine or some apple cider vinegar, if using. Vinegar is often used for fermented hot sauces as it increases the acidity, making the sauce more shelf stable. That said, I'd suggest keeping all blended hot sauces in the fridge as they can attract unwanted yeast.

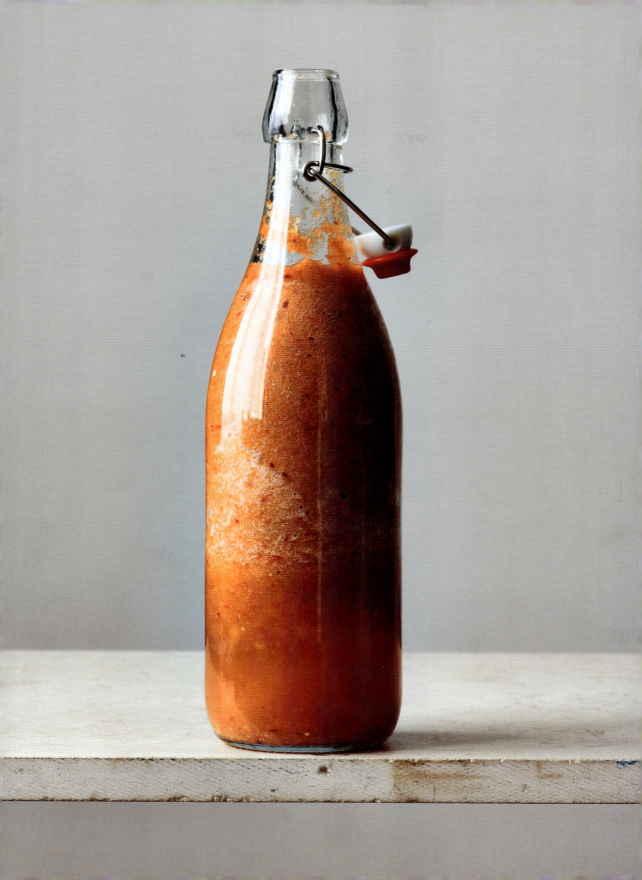

FENNEL, APPLE & CARAWAY SAUERKRAUT

Caraway is a typical flavor in traditional sauerkraut, but I think it really shines against the natural sweetness of fennel and apple. It's a nice twist on the classic and a welcome change from the usual cabbage-forward sauerkrauts. Enjoy this as you would any other sauerkraut; it works excellently in my Sauerkraut Latkes (see page 160).

PREP TIME: 15 MINUTES | FERMENTATION TIME: 2–5 WEEKS

Makes one 1-liter (1-quart) jar

600g (1lb 5oz) fennel
300g (10.5oz) apples (peel included)
measured salt: 2% of the total weight of above ingredients
1 tbsp caraway seeds

Thinly slice the fennel with a knife or mandoline and grate the apples.

In a large bowl, weigh these ingredients and calculate 2% of that total weight. This is the amount of salt you will need.

Add the salt to the fennel and apples and massage for 5–10 minutes, using a fair amount of pressure to optimize the creation of brine. If you do not see much brine, continue massaging and a pool of brine should appear.

Sprinkle the caraway seeds into the salted fennel and apples and mix thoroughly.

Decant into a jar and pack it down to ensure there are no air pockets in your sauerkraut, allowing the brine to gather on top of the apple and fennel. Use a food-safe fermentation weight to ensure everything is below the brine.

Cover the jar and leave it at room temperature and out of direct sunlight to ferment for 2–5 weeks. After 2 weeks, start tasting the sauerkraut. When you're pleased with the flavor, move it to the fridge where it will keep indefinitely.

CHIPOTLE & CARROT SAUERKRAUT

While carrots can be fermented in a wet brine—as seen in the Fermented Crudités on page 38—you can shred them and use the dry brining method to create a very different pickle. This is what I love about fermentation: Based on the vegetables you have on hand, you can extend their life in so many different ways.

This is a relatively simple one in terms of flavor: I've always found chipotle to lend both sweetness and spice, which works well with the natural sweetness from carrots, and there's a warming effect from the ginger. This ferment can sometimes be particularly active due to the sugar content of the carrots, so keep an eye on it, especially during the first week of fermentation.

This is excellent with chili or tacos, or, thanks to its bright color, as an addition to your next pickle platter.

PREP TIME: 15 MINUTES | FERMENTATION TIME: 2–5 WEEKS

Makes one 500-ml (1-pint) jar

- **450g (1lb) carrots, grated (peel included)**
- **15g (0.5oz) fresh ginger, peeled and grated**
- **measured salt: 2% of the total weight of above ingredients**
- **½ tsp chipotle chile flakes**

In a large bowl, weigh the carrots and ginger and calculate 2% of that total weight. This is the amount of salt you will need.

Add the salt to the bowl and massage the ingredients. Carrots generally emit a lot of water quickly, so will probably not require as much force or time as cabbage. Sprinkle in the chile flakes and mix to combine.

Decant into a jar and pack it down to ensure there are no air pockets in your sauerkraut, allowing the brine to gather on top of the carrots and ginger. Use a food-safe fermentation weight to ensure everything is below the brine.

Cover the jar and leave it at room temperature and out of direct sunlight to ferment for 2–5 weeks. After 2 weeks, start tasting the sauerkraut. When you're pleased with the flavor, move it to the fridge where it will keep indefinitely.

LACTOFERMENTATION

KIMCHI

On a sunny Mumbai weekend back in 2011, I set myself a mission to make kimchi, arguably one of the most quintessential Korean foods.

I had been living in Mumbai for a few months and once the dust had settled after my international move, it was time to set up my kitchen pantry. Coming from the States, I had been spoiled with accessible Korean grocery stores filled with large jars of affordable kimchi which, during my time in college, became one of my favorite foods to have around. My Korean American friends always knew which brands to buy when we made our monthly pilgrimage to the Asian supermarkets, or would fill our small fridge with containers of deliciously pungent kimchi brought from home, recipes passed down from grandparents to parents. Needless to say, I became a kimchi convert and soon found myself eating it alongside most dishes. I therefore never really had a reason to make kimchi from scratch. With ambitious naivety I traversed my local Mumbai markets (and the fancy overpriced expat-centric grocery store) to source all of the necessary ingredients. Finding the vegetables and aromatics was simple, but there was one fairly important element that I could not find: gochugaru chili flakes.

As it was my first time fermenting in Mumbai as well as making kimchi, I approached the process and recipe with rigidity. *Kimchi without gochugaru? Would that even be possible?* Little did I know that kimchi encompasses a broad diversity of techniques, including ones without gochugaru. Slightly defeated, I returned to my kitchen to rethink the plan. I rummaged through our cabinets and paused at my flatmate's metal masala dabba, or circular spice box. Staring back at me was red Kashmiri chili powder. Bright red, slightly fruity, and not excessively spicy, this alternative was the final puzzle piece and by day's end I had two jars of kimchi bubbling away in the heat of the Mumbai summer. Remember, fermentation is faster in warmer environments.

India was perhaps a surprising location to set out on my kimchi-making journey. But on reflection, it was a prime example of how location and ingredient accessibility not only influence a recipe but also drive innovation, and ultimately sustain food traditions. As I learned more about kimchi, and dived deeper into this fantastic Korean ferment, I was inspired to learn about regional variations, speaking to my Korean American friends who told me about their family recipes: shortcuts incorporated by busy parents and adaptations for American palates. Raw oysters added for an umami sweetness which celebrated proximity to the Korean coasts just as halmeoni (grandmother) made. Or even how kimchi evolved throughout history as people migrated or were displaced, as with Morkovcha (see page 70), a Central Asian/Eastern European version created by Koreans in the 1930s. I also saw this evolution of techniques and flavors in Indian-style kimchi, a vinegar-based slaw-like salad, often served as a starter in East Asian restaurants in Mumbai in the early 2010s.

While I now have a steady supply of gochugaru chili flakes, the memory of first making kimchi in Mumbai has been a constant source of creativity in how I approach preservation at home. I would now argue that gochugaru is a non-negotiable ingredient when making standard varieties of kimchi, but I do believe there are endless possibilities in both approach and application which still honor traditional methods, as you'll see in some of the recipes that follow.

With this lens, I challenge you to apply these traditions to new ingredients, and the produce you have at home. Lactofermentation is the preservation method here, but I want to highlight that not only can kimchi be made with unique aromatics and flavorings, but that kimchi itself is an evolving ingredient. Most of my recipes require a fairly short period of fermentation at room temperature before moving the kimchi to the fridge for both longer-term storage and to slow down the fermentation. I prefer the taste and texture of fresher kimchi, but older and more fermented kimchi has its place: You may enjoy the tangier flavors, especially when served on a pickle platter alongside fresher varieties, and it's also a flavor powerhouse in your cooking, which I'll dive into with some of my favorite recipes later in the book.

The beautiful history of kimchi acts as a reminder that all these preservation techniques can evolve based on preference, locality, and accessibility, which is true of so many other diasporic food traditions. And who knows, maybe one day your grandchildren will reminisce about the kimchi they grew up with: a celebration of exchange, with people and the memories they carry, as well as the physical locations that have grounded these practices.

KIMCHI 101

I make kimchi at least once a month—and often without a recipe. Some will have more aromatics in the form of garlic, ginger, and onion, all of which can vary in terms of heat or spice level. I may swap sugar for honey, a cheong (see pages 142–147), or additional fruit (apple and pear are my preferences). And in terms of salt and umami, I tend to rotate between fish sauce, miso, and soy sauce.

There is significant variation within this traditional ferment based on traditions, process, and access, but below is my go-to recipe for kimchi—perhaps the most "traditional" in terms of process and ingredients. I expect with practice your own kimchi will evolve and develop based on your own taste and preferences.

PREP TIME: 30 MINUTES + 1 hour salting
FERMENTATION TIME: 2–10 DAYS

Makes one 1-liter (1-quart) jar

- 500g (1lb 2oz) napa cabbage
- 100g (3.5oz) carrot, peeled and julienned
- 100g (3.5oz) daikon radish (mooli), julienned
- measured salt: 3% of the total weight of above ingredients
- 3 green onions, trimmed and thinly sliced

FOR THE RICE PORRIDGE

- 1½ tsp glutinous rice flour
- 1 tbsp sugar

Wash and core the cabbage—I like to use as much of the cabbage as possible. Depending on the size, I generally cut it into quarters or eighths lengthwise and then chop it into large bite-size pieces. Put the chopped cabbage into a large bowl, along with the carrot and daikon.

Weigh the vegetables and calculate 3% of the total weight. This is the amount of salt you will need.

Sprinkle the salt onto the prepared vegetables and massage it in for 5–10 minutes to start the natural brining process in which water is drawn out from the vegetables. Leave the vegetables to salt for 1 hour, giving them a squeeze and a flip halfway to ensure all the cabbage has wilted and there's brine at the bottom of the bowl.

While the vegetables are salting, make the rice porridge: Put the glutinous rice flour and 120ml (½ cup) water in a small saucepan over a low heat, and whisk to prevent the flour from clumping. Once the water starts to warm up, the mixture will quickly thicken. Whisk in the sugar, then remove the rice porridge from the heat and cool to room temperature.

FOR THE PASTE

50g (1.75oz) apple (about ½ apple), peeled and roughly chopped

50g (1.75oz) onion (about ½ onion), peeled and roughly chopped

15g (0.5oz) garlic (about 3 cloves), peeled and roughly chopped

15g (0.5oz) fresh ginger, peeled and roughly chopped

2 tbsp fish sauce

25g (1oz) coarse gochugaru

SPECIAL EQUIPMENT: food processor

To make the paste, put the chopped apple in a food processor, along with the onion, garlic, ginger, fish sauce, and gochugaru. Blitz to a smooth, thick paste which will loosen as we assemble the kimchi.

After 1 hour, rinse the salted vegetables with fresh water and squeeze out any residual water. The vegetables should all be rather pliable.

In a large bowl, combine the salted and rinsed vegetables, rice porridge, and paste. Stir in the green onions. Mix thoroughly and put it into a clean glass jar. Pack everything down to minimize air pockets.

Ferment at room temperature for a minimum of 2 days and up to 10 days; the flavors will mellow with time, so taste it daily to learn how it ferments in your environment. Once you're pleased with the sourness, move it to the fridge where it will keep indefinitely.

A few notes:

— **Rice porridge** is a traditional element in the kimchi paste but I know many Koreans of the diaspora who do not include this or replace it with whizzed up leftover rice or even boiled and mashed potatoes. This may sound odd but it makes sense if you understand the role rice porridge plays here: It not only adds texture to the paste, making it easier to adhere to the cabbage leaves, but it also acts as an additional source of food for the bacteria.

— In terms of **umami**, my recipe uses only fish sauce, but many also include salted shrimp as an additional source of umami; I've always struggled with finding the right ones so tend to omit this. If you can get them easily, definitely try it out. Vegetarian alternatives include miso, plant-based fish sauce, or soy sauce.

— Most recipes for cabbage-based kimchi require you to **rinse the salt off** before adding the paste. This may surprise you given that this is lactofermentation and therefore requires salt for its safe preservation. That said, the fish sauce or miso in the paste provides sufficient salt for safe fermentation. If you're interested in seeing how the end product differs, check out the process for my Corner Store Kimchi (see page 58), which incorporates the salty brine into the kimchi.

— **Use your hands!** I use my hands when making cabbage-based kimchi to ensure the paste is adequately mixed throughout the vegetables, which works better than a spoon in my opinion. Remember that fermentation should be a sensory experience, so get involved!

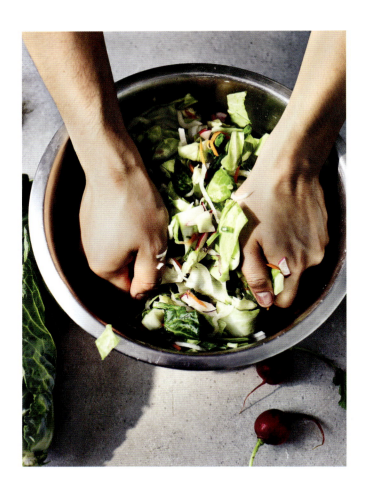
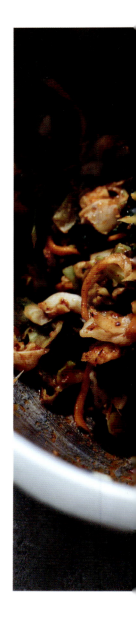

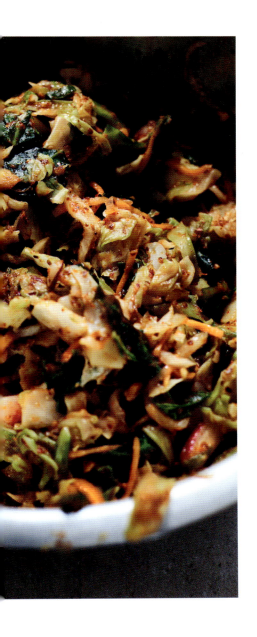
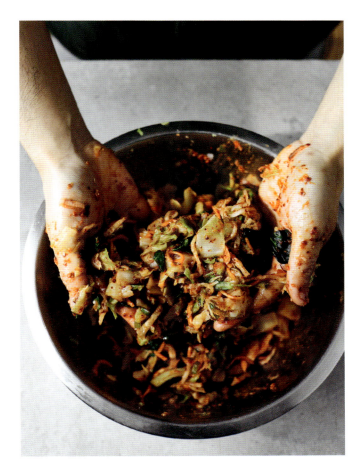

CORNER STORE KIMCHI

This corner store kimchi is my go-to recipe when I'm itching for my kimchi fix but can't get to specialty stores. Here, I swap napa cabbage and daikon radish (mooli) for sweetheart (hispi) cabbage and small red radishes, both ingredients I can find at my local store. And leaning even further into the theme of convenience and low-waste, I like to throw both the green onion whites and roots into the paste—just make sure that the roots are cleaned of any dirt.

The process is fairly similar to my basic kimchi (see page 54) with some notable changes: no rice porridge; no need to rinse the cabbage—I use some of the salted brine to act as both safeguard and fermentation accelerator; and I use miso instead of the more commonly used fish sauce and/or shrimp paste as a source of umami and salt. So yes, it's plant-based, and a good entry-level ferment. *See step-by-step images on pages 56–57.*

PREP TIME: 30 MINUTES + 1 hour salting | FERMENTATION TIME: 2–10 DAYS

Makes one 1-liter (1-quart) jar

500g (1lb 2oz) sweetheart (hispi) cabbage, halved

100g (3.5oz) carrot, peeled and grated or julienned

100g (3.5oz) red radishes, quartered

measured salt: 3% of the total weight of above ingredients

FOR THE PASTE

3 green onions, greens, whites, and roots separated

15g (0.5oz) garlic (about 3 cloves), peeled and roughly chopped

15g (0.5oz) fresh ginger, peeled and roughly chopped

50g (1.75oz) apple (about ½ apple), roughly chopped (peel included)

1 tbsp sugar

25g (1oz) coarse gochugaru

1 tbsp red miso

SPECIAL EQUIPMENT: food processor

Shred the cabbage into roughly 1cm (½in) pieces using a sharp knife. Place the shredded cabbage in a bowl with the carrot and radishes and calculate 3% of the total weight. This is the amount of salt you will need.

Add the salt to the vegetables and massage it in for 5–10 minutes to start the natural brining process. Leave the vegetables to salt for 1 hour, giving them a squeeze and a flip halfway to ensure all the cabbage has wilted and there's brine at the bottom of the bowl.

While the vegetables are salting, prepare the paste by blitzing the white part and cleaned roots of the green onions (reserving the greens) in a food processor with the rest of the ingredients until it becomes a thick paste.

After 1 hour, squeeze the vegetables and reserve the brine. Thinly slice the green onion greens. Combine the squeezed cabbage, carrot, and radishes with the green onion greens and the paste in a large bowl. Add 150ml (½ cup plus 2 tablespoons) of the reserved brine and mix thoroughly. Put it into a clean glass jar and to minimize air pockets.

Ferment at room temperature for a minimum of 2 days and up to 10 days; the flavors will mellow with time, so taste it daily. Once you're pleased with the sourness, move it to the fridge where it will keep indefinitely.

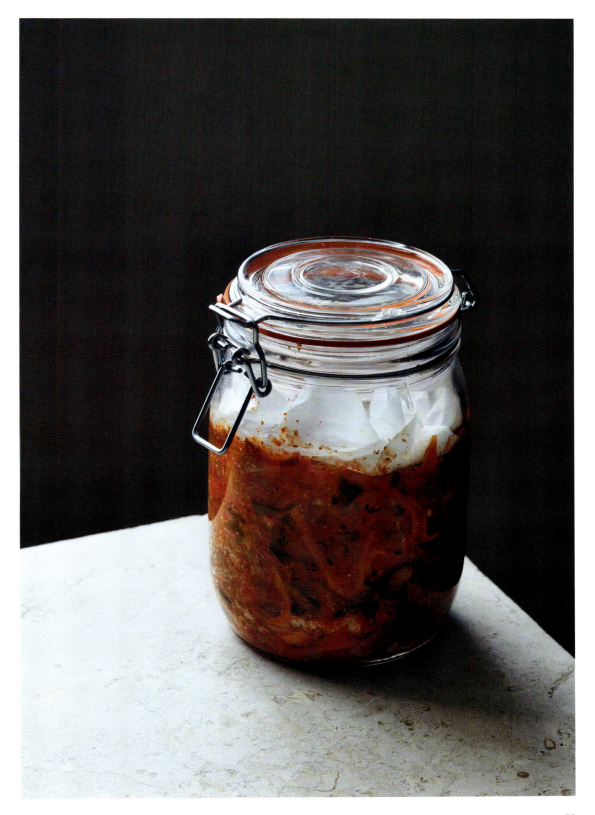

WATERMELON RIND KIMCHI

Fermenting seasonally is a joy, and a signifier for the passage of time. I look forward to watermelon season more for the rind than for the fruit itself. I'm sure many of you compost the rind, but I challenge you to view it as its own ingredient, full of potential and a way to reduce waste in your kitchen.

I compare watermelon rind to daikon radish (mooli) in both texture and application. However, I've realized that watermelons are not created equal: Some have rather thick skin and an even thicker rind, which may mean a vegetable peeler is insufficient to produce a palatably textured rind. You're aiming for a texture that is not too hard, similar to what you'd expect from daikon radish, so you may need to trim more from the outer surface with a knife to produce the correct texture, pre-fermentation. If the rind is too hard, it will not ferment as effectively and may require more time.

This is inspired by daikon radish kimchi, called kkakdugi. But leaning into the watermelon theme, I've incorporated its juice and flesh into the paste, as well as black sesame seeds to act as a visual play on the fruit's seeds. Use the remaining watermelon flesh to flavor kombucha or enjoy it as it is with Kimchi Sprinkles (see page 76).

PREP TIME: 15 MINUTES + 1 hour salting | FERMENTATION TIME: 2–3 DAYS

Makes one 500-ml (1-pint) jar

- 500g (1lb 2oz) watermelon rind (the rind from roughly 1 watermelon), 2 tbsp flesh reserved
- measured salt: 2% of the total weight of the rind
- 10g (0.33oz) garlic (1–2 cloves), peeled and grated
- 10g (0.33oz) fresh ginger, peeled and grated
- 1 tbsp apple cider vinegar
- 2 tbsp coarse gochugaru
- 2 tbsp watermelon juice
- 1 tsp fish sauce
- 2 tsp black sesame seeds

Using a vegetable peeler, peel your watermelon rind and scoop out any flesh and juice. Cut the rind into small cubes (about 1.5cm/⅔in) and put them into a bowl.

Weigh the watermelon rind and calculate 2% of the weight. This is the amount of salt you will need. Sprinkle the salt over the rind and leave to salt for 1 hour, mixing halfway to ensure even salt coverage.

After 1 hour, add the reserved watermelon flesh and all the remaining ingredients to the bowl and give everything a good mix. Decant it into a clean glass jar, ensuring that all of the watermelon rind is submerged in the brine.

Ferment at room temperature for 2 days, then move it to the fridge, where it will keep indefinitely; that said, I prefer this one when it's fresher.

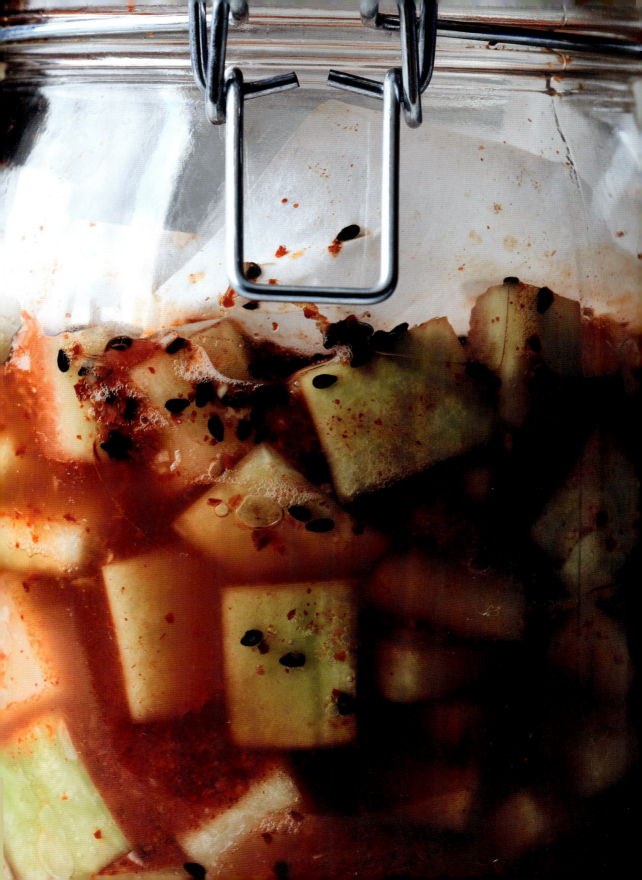

CUCUMBER SNAKE-CUT KIMCHI

Oisobagi (or Korean stuffed cucumber kimchi) is a favorite in my home. Traditionally, small cucumbers are quartered and stuffed with the kimchi paste. However, in this version I explore how surface area can impact a pickle. How a vegetable is processed directly affects its flavor. This is true for all forms of kitchen sorcery, but in pickling and fermentation, increasing surface area not only accelerates the removal of excess water, but also allows the vegetable to absorb flavor more efficiently.

In Japanese, this preparation is called "snake belly cut" or jabara-giri: The cucumber is scored diagonally on both sides, producing an accordion-like effect. As the cucumber softens, thanks to the salt, it becomes flexible and rather snake-like (hence the name). This is not only very cool and fun—and who doesn't love a wow factor with their pickle offerings—but is also a lesson on the importance of surface area when pickling. And for this reason, I encourage you to start eating these immediately and note how the flavors and textures evolve. In fact, they are delicious when freshly made and can be eaten much like a salad. You may find that you eat them all up even before they start fermenting properly! *See photos on pages 64–65.*

PREP TIME: 15 MINUTES + 30 minutes salting
FERMENTATION TIME: 1 DAY

MAKES 450G (1LB)

450g (1lb) small cucumbers

measured salt: 3% of the total weight of the cucumbers

1 carrot, peeled and julienned

6 green onions, trimmed and thinly sliced

FOR THE PASTE

10g (0.33oz) garlic (1–2 cloves), peeled and grated

10g (0.33oz) fresh ginger, peeled and grated

60ml (¼ cup) fish sauce

3 tbsp coarse gochugaru

1½ tsp sugar

1½ tsp sesame seeds

Prepare the cucumbers by trimming off both ends, then start on the snake belly cut: Lay each cucumber on a cutting board between two disposable chopsticks and slice it at an angle as thinly as possible (about 3mm/⅛in) against the chopsticks so you do not cut all the way through the cucumber. When you have sliced along the length of the cucumber, flip it over and repeat the process.

When you have cut all the cucumbers in this way, weigh them and calculate 3% of the total weight. This is the amount of salt you will need.

Put the cut cucumbers into a large bowl and sprinkle the salt over them. Use your hands to gently rub each cucumber with the salt; aim to work the salt evenly throughout the cucumbers, including through the incisions. Leave to salt for 30 minutes, giving the cucumbers an occasional mix.

While the cucumbers are salting, make the paste by combining all of the ingredients in a small bowl.

After 30 minutes, rinse the cucumbers with fresh water and give them a light squeeze to remove residual moisture. Put them into a large bowl, add the carrots, paste, and green onions and mix well.

Put everything into a jar or covered food-safe container and ferment at room temperature for up to 1 day, then move it to the fridge for long-term storage. The snake-cut cucumbers will continue to emit water, so aim to eat them within a few weeks.

How can I use my kimchi brine?

Don't throw away all that flavor and instead use it in any of the following ways:

—If it's not too diluted, use it as a source of flavor for a quick pickle or to marinate vegetables or protein (as in the Kimchi-Brined Fried Chicken on page 218).

—Use it for dressings, mixed into aiolis, or to loosen sauces with some additional acidity and heat (see the Ten-Minute Miso Peanut Butter Kimchi Noodles on page 212).

—Use it as a brine shot for a pickle platter or add it to cocktails (see the Kimchi Bloody Mary on page 256).

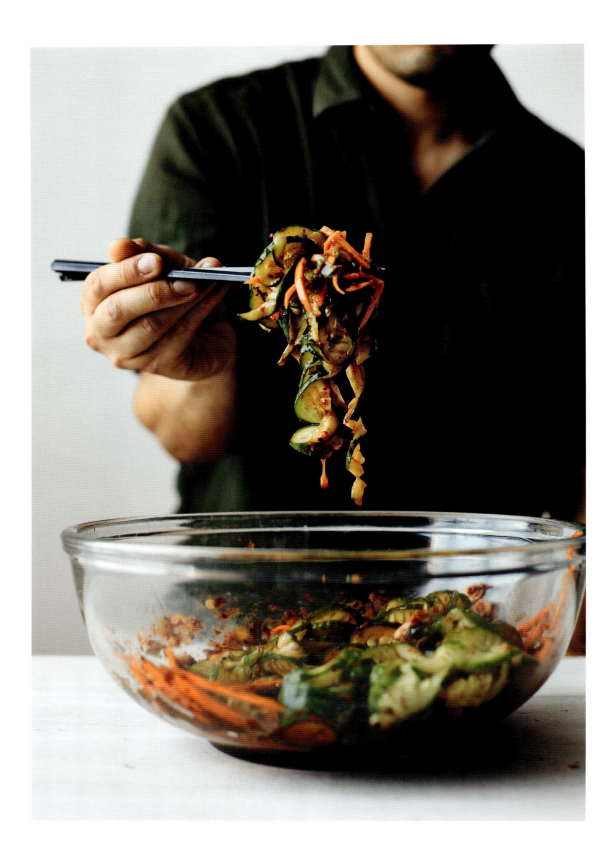

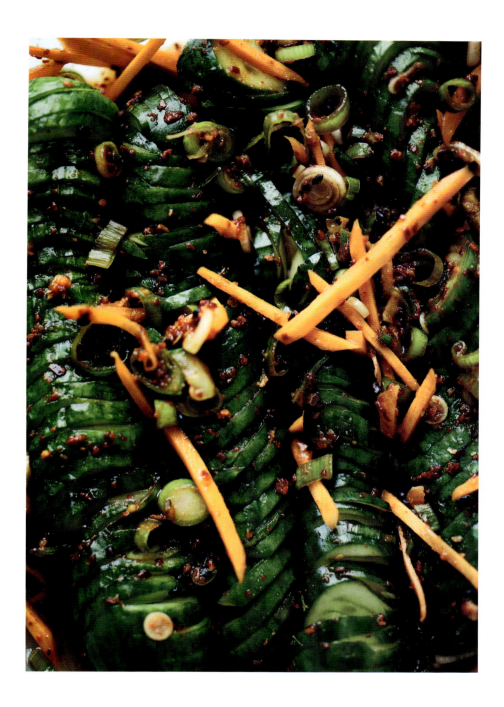

CHERRY TOMATO KIMCHI

Is this kimchi? Some may say no since there's no obvious fermentation and it's eaten so soon after making, but what makes a kimchi a kimchi? Perhaps this is more accurately termed a side dish with kimchi flavorings, but I tend to view kimchi—and all forms of preservation—as a spectrum. As soon as you cut the tomatoes and allow the ingredients to mingle, the process of preservation begins: Salt draws out moisture and the tomatoes absorb the flavors of the aromatics, fermented fish sauce, and kombucha citrus syrup.

Tomatoes have a high water content so this is best eaten within a few days as it tends to dilute over time. It's delicious as is but also great thrown into salads, stir-fries, or really any dish where tomatoes are called for—however, I think it is best when served with my Kimchi-Brined Fried Chicken (see page 218).

PREP TIME: 10 MINUTES + 10 minutes salting
WAIT TIME: 1 HOUR

Makes one 500-ml (1-pint) jar

- 450g (1lb) cherry tomatoes, halved
- ½ tsp salt
- 1 garlic clove, peeled and grated
- 1 tbsp lemon juice
- 4 green onions, green part only, sliced
- 1 tbsp fish sauce
- 1 tbsp Kombucha Citrus Syrup (see page 138) or honey
- 1 tsp sugar
- 1 tbsp coarse gochugaru

Put the cherry tomatoes in a bowl and sprinkle with the salt to draw out excess moisture. Let this stand for 10 minutes.

Mix the garlic with the lemon juice and set aside for a few minutes to soften the garlic's intensity.

Add the garlic and lemon juice to the tomatoes, along with all of the other ingredients. Give them a mix—no need to be gentle, as the juices from the tomatoes are part of the brine.

Marinate for around 1 hour at room temperature before digging in.

Keep this in the fridge in an airtight container; it is best consumed within a week.

BRUSSELS SPROUT & CRANBERRY KIMCHI

As the days grow shorter and autumn turns to winter, this seasonal kimchi is the perfect addition to your festive feasts. While I'd argue that any pickle or ferment would be a welcome addition to any meal, there's something about rich dishes in cold weather that just cry out for a zingy accompaniment.

Brussels sprouts and cranberries are two of the ingredients we generally associate with this time of the year, so combining them for a festive kimchi makes a lot of sense, doesn't it? The shredded brussels sprouts mimic the surface area of shredded cabbage and will therefore increase the output of brine. Dried cranberries add a source of sugar—both blended into the paste and left whole in the kimchi itself. Taste this regularly and you'll observe how the dried fruit imparts its natural sweetness. I think this one gets better with age, which is a departure from my general preference for freshly made kimchi. Enjoy this kimchi any way you like, but it is particularly good in a grilled cheese with all the best festive leftovers!

PREP TIME: 20 MINUTES + 1–3 hours salting
FERMENTATION TIME: 5–7 DAYS

Makes one 500-ml (1-pint) jar

- 300g (10.5oz) brussels sprouts, trimmed and shredded
- measured salt: 3% of the total weight of the sprouts
- 20g (0.75oz) dried cranberries

FOR THE PASTE

- 20g (0.75oz) garlic (about 3–4 cloves), peeled and grated
- 20g (0.75oz) fresh ginger, peeled and grated
- 20g (0.75oz) coarse gochugaru
- 40g (1.5oz) dried cranberries
- 40g (1.5oz) apple, roughly chopped (peel included)
- 1½ tsp fish sauce or red miso

SPECIAL EQUIPMENT: food processor

Prepare the brussels sprouts and weigh them. Calculate 3% of the weight. This is the amount of salt you will need. Put the shredded brussels sprouts into a bowl, sprinkle with the salt, and give this a thorough mix with your hands to ensure the salt is evenly distributed. Leave to salt for at least 1 hour, or up to 3 hours, mixing every 30 minutes. During this time, the brussels sprouts should emit brine as they wilt.

While the brussels sprouts are salting, make the paste: Put all of the ingredients into a food processor with 1 tablespoon of water and blitz.

When the brussels sprouts have softened and emitted brine, add the paste to the bowl, along with the whole cranberries, and mix thoroughly.

Pack the kimchi into a jar, pressing down to minimize air pockets and ensuring that everything is below the brine.

Ferment at room temperature for 5–7 days; start tasting after 5 days and when you're happy with the flavor, move it to the fridge where it will keep indefinitely.

MORKOVCHA

Morkovcha is a version of kimchi found throughout post-Soviet countries in Eastern Europe, originated by displaced Korean populations known as the Koryo-saram. When you make this, you'll find some similarities with kimchi, although it's ultimately very different in both ingredients and process. I wanted to include this recipe as it reflects a time and place the way that recipes can evolve due to displacement and accessibility—themes close to my own family history.

Napa cabbages weren't readily available to the Koryo-saram, so carrots were swapped in for the key ingredient. Even the name of this dish signals this confluence of cultures and traditions, morkovcha being a combination of the Russian word for carrot (*morkov*) and the Korean word for a salad-type dish (*chae*). As the name suggests, treat this more as a salad and each time you eat it—as a side dish or alongside other pickles—remember its origin and how access (or lack thereof) leads to innovation and creativity in food.

PREP TIME: 15 MINUTES | WAIT TIME: 5 HOURS

Makes one 500-ml (1-pint) jar

- 500g (1lb 2oz) carrots, peeled and julienned (or grated)
- ½ tsp ground coriander
- ½ tsp paprika
- 1 tsp coarse gochugaru
- ½ tsp ground black pepper
- 1 tsp salt
- 1 tsp sugar
- 2 tbsp vinegar (white wine, rice wine, or my favorite, apple cider vinegar)
- 4 garlic cloves, finely chopped
- 3 tbsp vegetable oil
- 1 tsp white sesame seeds
- handful of fresh cilantro, finely chopped

Put the carrots in a large bowl and mix in all of the dried spices, sugar, and vinegar. Put the garlic on top of the carrot mixture—do not mix this in.

Heat the oil in a frying pan over a medium heat until smoking and pour over the garlic, thereby tempering it. Mix everything together and then add the sesame seeds and cilantro. Enjoy this immediately (or after a few hours in the fridge). It is best consumed within a week.

FENNEL & TURMERIC KIMCHI

My nostalgic take on Indian-style kimchi

This is the love child of the two varieties of kimchi referenced in the introduction to this section: the first kimchi I ever made (with some ingredients swapped out due to what I had access to when living in Mumbai) and the seemingly ubiquitous kimchi-like salad I enjoyed in East Asian restaurants in Mumbai, circa 2012.

In terms of process and flavor profile, this is not so far outside the realm of kimchi: gently fermented, cabbage-based, and with the familiar aromatics. What is slightly unorthodox, however, is the addition of vinegar; it is not an ingredient I'd usually include when making kimchi, but it adds a fruity acidity and is an homage to those kimchi-like salads. And of course the spices lean into a South Asian palate: Kashmiri chili instead of gochugaru for heat, turmeric for color, and fennel seed—since it's one of my favorite spices. This is delicious served with a dash of toasted sesame oil. *See photos on page 72-73.*

PREP TIME: 15 MINUTES + 2-3 hours salting
FERMENTATION TIME: 24 HOURS

Makes one 1-liter (1-quart) jar

- 750g (1lb 10oz) white cabbage, core removed, cut into bite-size pieces
- measured salt: 3% of the total weight of the cabbage
- 20g (0.75oz) fresh ginger, peeled and finely chopped
- 20g (0.75oz) garlic (about 3-4 cloves), peeled and finely chopped
- 1 tbsp light soy sauce
- 1 tbsp apple cider vinegar
- 2 tsp sugar
- 1 tsp Kashmiri chili powder
- 1 tsp fennel seeds
- 1 tsp ground turmeric
- 3 green onions, trimmed and thinly sliced

Weigh the prepared cabbage and calculate 3% of the weight. This is the amount of salt you will need.

Put the cabbage in a mixing bowl and mix in the salt. Give the cabbage a massage for 5-10 minutes and leave to salt at room temperature for 2-3 hours, squeezing and flipping it every 30 minutes, until the cabbage has wilted and brine has gathered at the bottom of the bowl.

Rinse the cabbage with fresh water and squeeze out as much liquid as possible. Put the washed and drained cabbage into a bowl, add all the remaining ingredients, and mix thoroughly.

Decant into a jar. Use force to pack the cabbage into the jar to ensure the brine covers the bulk of the cabbage. Leave at room temperature for 24 hours and then move to the fridge; it is best consumed within a few weeks.

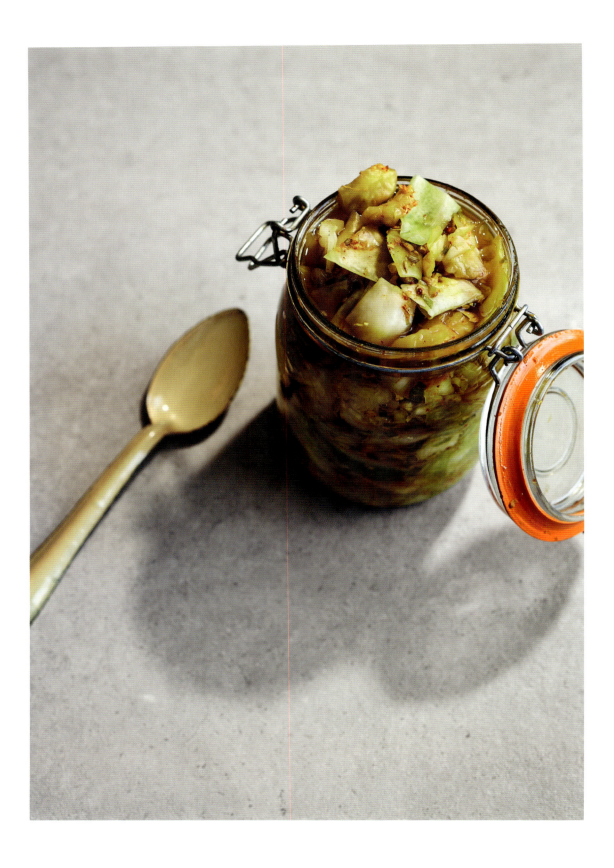

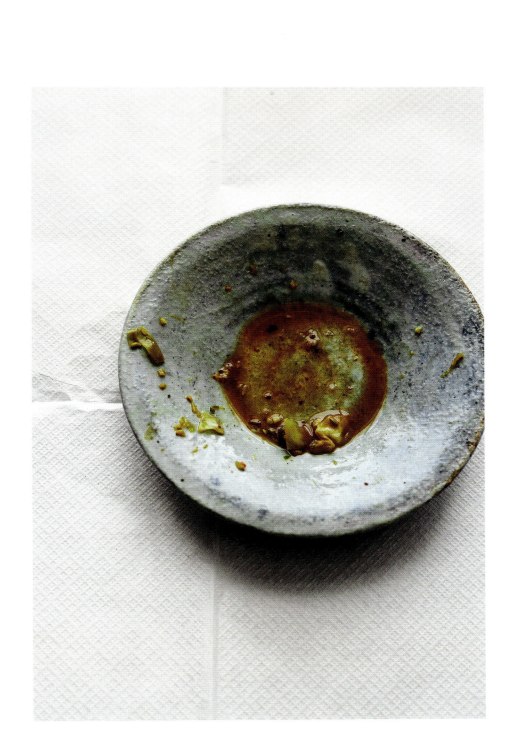

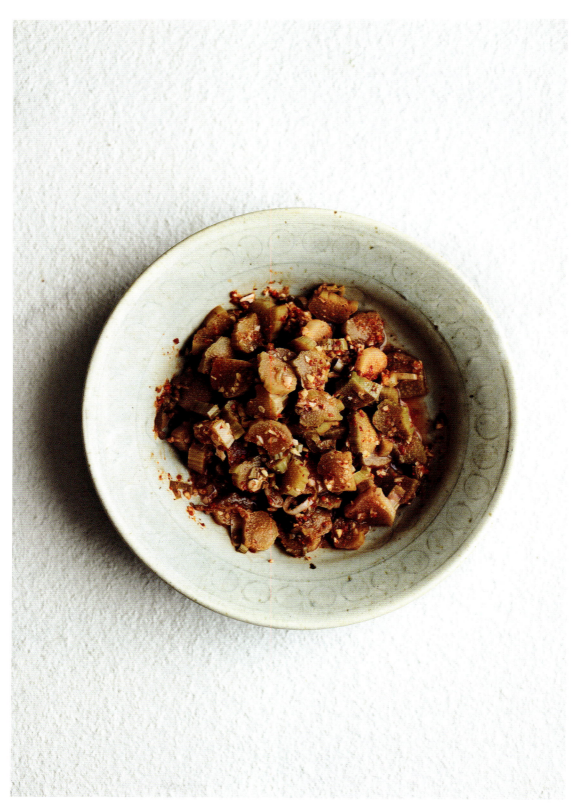

RHUBARB KIMCHI

You'll find that rhubarb comes up a few times in this book and it's honestly because, of all the seasonal produce to look forward to, I get most excited about rhubarb. I even have two fairly unproductive but healthy rhubarb plants in my back garden, and while I haven't grown enough to make the recipe below with home-grown rhubarb, I dream of the day I'll harvest enough to make this special seasonal kimchi.

I think this kimchi is best eaten fresh, usually after two days depending on how warm your kitchen is; it retains the crunch and it's objectively bright, the sourness balancing nicely against the citric sumac and orange.

Eat this kimchi as you would eat any pickle. Fairly versatile, its flavors jiving with most cuisines, it demands attention on a cheese platter. As it ages, the rhubarb loses its structure, but then you're left with the perfect accompaniment to a hot bowl of freshly cooked rice, somewhat reminding me of a Japanese salted and pickled plum (umeboshi).

PREP TIME: 20 MINUTES | FERMENTATION TIME: 2 DAYS

Makes one 500-ml (1-pint) jar

- 450g (1lb) rhubarb, trimmed and cut into 5mm-thick (¼in) slices
- measured salt: 2% of the total weight of the rhubarb
- 2 green onions, trimmed and thinly sliced

FOR THE PASTE

- 10g (0.33oz) fresh ginger, peeled and finely chopped
- 10g (0.33oz) garlic (about 1–2 cloves), peeled and finely chopped
- 10g (0.33oz) coarse gochugaru
- 1 tsp sumac
- zest of 1 orange
- 2 tbsp orange juice

SPECIAL EQUIPMENT: food processor (optional)

Weigh the prepared rhubarb and calculate 2% of the weight. This is the amount of salt you'll need.
Put the chopped rhubarb in a large bowl, sprinkle with the salt, and give it a thorough mix. Let it stand for 10 minutes.
 While the rhubarb is salting, make the paste: Put all of the ingredients into a food processor and blitz until finely chopped and combined. As it's a small amount of paste, you can also do this by hand.
 Add the paste and the sliced green onions to the bowl and mix everything together.
 Decant the kimchi into a jar. Use force to pack the rhubarb into the jar to ensure the brine covers the bulk of the rhubarb. Leave at room temperature for 2 days (or longer); start tasting after 2 days and when you're happy with the flavor, move it to the fridge where it will keep indefinitely, but it is best consumed within a month if you want to maintain its texture.

KIMCHI SPRINKLES

Dehydrating fermented vegetables—from kimchi to sauerkraut—is not only an excellent way to breathe new life into your over-fermented pickles that may be slightly past their prime, but a way to transform them into a new ingredient. Cooking with ferments, as I'll explore later in the book, is a fantastic way to immediately add flavor and complexity and, as expected, this becomes even further magnified when dehydrated. In the case of kimchi, you're left with an intensely savory and tangy item which is equal parts ingredient and treat.

It makes a really good jerky-like beer snack as is but I find it most versatile in my home cooking when it's blitzed in a food processor. It can be used as a garnish on rice (similar to a Japanese furikake), added to salads, tossed into popcorn (an all-time favorite), or used as a source of flavor and texture in miso soups (or in my Sweet Pickle Tuna Summer Rolls, which you can find on page 205).

I haven't given a specific quantity because this can be done with any amount of kimchi. However, as I aim to be efficient with my oven usage, I generally tend to do larger batches of kimchi as I get through these sprinkles quickly. For reference, in a recent batch, I started off with 800g (1.75lbs) of kimchi, and after dehydrating, ended up with 100g (3.5oz). *See photo on pages 78–79.*

PREP TIME: 10 MINUTES | COOK TIME: up to 7 HOURS

kimchi (I find that cabbage-forward varieties of kimchi work best. However, any kimchi will technically work—you will just need to adjust the dehydrating time as some vegetables have a higher water content and will therefore require more time)

SPECIAL EQUIPMENT: food dehydrator (optional); food processor or blender

Line a baking sheet with parchment paper. Squeeze your kimchi, reserving its brine for a different use, such as the Kimchi-Brined Fried Chicken (see page 218) or Kimchi Bloody Mary (see page 256). If the kimchi you are using is particularly large, chop it up as increasing surface area will speed up the dehydration.

Spread the squeezed-out kimchi on the lined baking sheet in a single layer, turn on your oven to 350°F (180°C) and dehydrate for around 7 hours. Check the kimchi every hour or so, and remove it from the oven once it's fully dehydrated. The total time in the oven may differ based on the kimchi you're using and its water content. Due to the low temperature there's very little risk of anything burning, but keep a watchful eye during this process. You could also use a food dehydrator to dehydrate the kimchi.

Once fully dehydrated, move the kimchi (and all of the delicious small bits—use a metal spatula to scrape the baking sheet) into a food processor or blender and blitz to your desired size. I generally keep the sprinkles rather coarse as I find them the most versatile. They can always be blitzed further and passed through a fine mesh strainer to make a powdered form.

If you're planning on using this primarily for savory food applications, you could add sesame seeds for additional crunch.

Keep this in an airtight container and it should last up to a year at room temperature—but I guarantee you'll get through it before then!

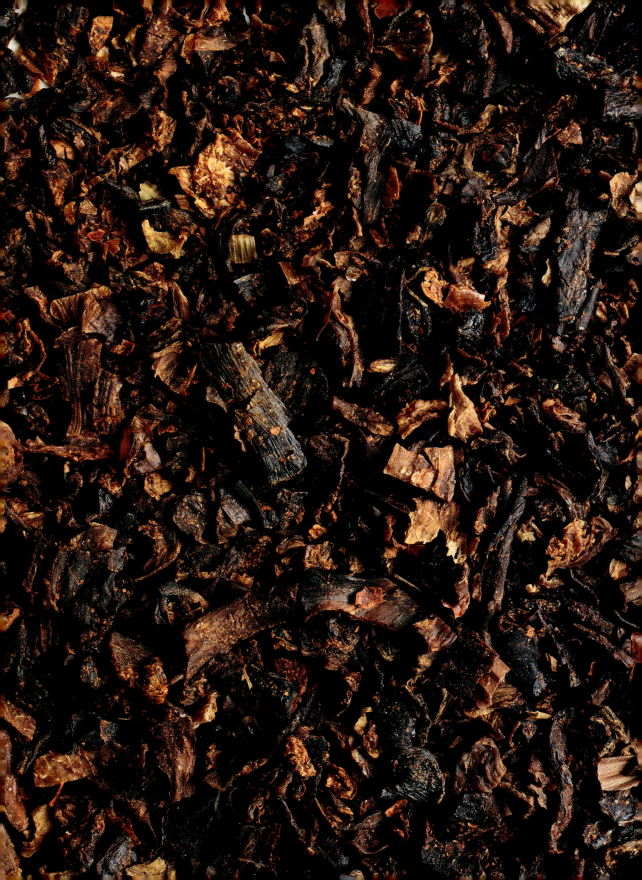

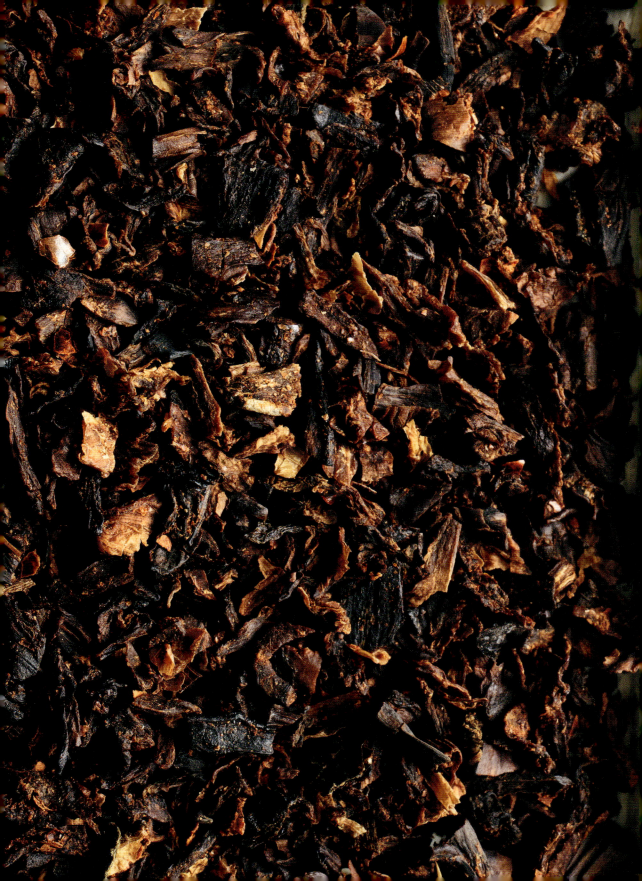

MISO

My deepest and oldest sense memories are the tastes and smells of Japanese food.

My love of Japanese food may seem natural, given my name, but my family's story is anything but straightforward. My great-grandparents immigrated to the USA in the 1880s and with a family history of over 140 years in the USA, I often struggled with questions about inclusion.

I grew up in a predominantly white neighborhood and was often one of only a handful of East Asians in my school. Consequently, I had the tiring task of repeatedly explaining who I was and where I was from (*no, really from*) and creating a space for myself. Will I always be labeled as a foreigner? Or will my merit justify a seat at the table, furthering the model minority myth? And as a result, will I always just be an "other"? While these are feelings I'm constantly grappling with as a Japanese American in London, the living definition of a third-culture adult, food is what has grounded me and provided a sense of belonging as my concept of home has evolved.

My grandmothers both had innate abilities to balance flavors in the kitchen, and they both taught me of the "*sa shi su se so*" of Japanese cooking. These letters each symbolize a fundamental element: *sa* for sugar, *shi* for salt, *su* for rice vinegar, *se* for shoyu (Japanese soy sauce), and *so* for miso. Of these five fundamental Japanese ingredients, three are fermented ingredients, and perhaps the one most unique to my ancestral home is miso, a fermented paste, most often made with soybeans.

I have countless memories of miso that touch on all of the senses: the sizzle of miso-glazed eggplant on my dad's barbecue, caramelized in gradient shades of brown; large vats of miso soup at my Buddhist temple, tofu and green onion dancing to the rhythm of a slow and steady simmer; and the earthy sweet scent of miso guiding me to that next bite, umami rich and satisfying.

My family did not make their own miso as we had plenty of options from our local Japanese stores. I think my grandparents would all find it rather humorous that their grandson is now making miso on a regular basis, but displacement is a common ingredient to many immigrant stories, and the nostalgic flavors of home serve as a tangible reminder of our origins.

I was raised a Buddhist and it was really through fermentation, and specifically making miso, that I have found meaning in its teachings of impermanence, patience, and letting go, as well as an acknowledgment and celebration of the passage of time. When I first saw my parents after the pandemic, I spent a lazy Sunday afternoon making miso with them. We sat around the dining room table, immersed in conversation, the microbes from our hands coming together in communion as we mashed soybeans and koji, and packed the miso into two jars: one for me, and one for my parents to be enjoyed in six months' time in Chicago. It was a really special moment and a true snapshot of us as parents and son; a tangible remembrance of our time together in the form of a creation that will continue to evolve, as one often does in life. A few other examples include the miso from the first workshop I taught, or the first experimental batch I made in Mumbai, which gave me the confidence to innovate and allowed me to challenge my assumptions about what miso is and can be.

Miso can be a long fermentation project, especially when compared to others in this book. You must trust the process and observe—almost in a meditative way—how miso evolves as it ferments: the colors darkening with age, tamari liquid pooling at the top, course-correcting as needed based on what you see, smell, and taste.

Above all, view miso as a spectrum of umami richness, as all accessible varieties are made of the same core four elements:

— **Soybeans:** the traditional bean and protein source for miso; however, they can be swapped for other legumes (such as chickpeas, lima beans, or lentils), or different ingredients entirely (such as butternut squash or beet, as shown later in this section).

— **Koji:** the name interchangeably used for both the fungus, *Aspergillus oryzae*, and rice (or other grains such as barley or soybeans) that has been inoculated with this fungus. Koji is packed with enzymes that break down complex carbohydrates and proteins into simple sugars and amino acids.

Steamed grains (most commonly rice) are inoculated with *Aspergillus oryzae* spores, referred to as a koji starter. The grains are incubated in a high humidity environment and kept at a stable warm temperature of 80–95°F (27–35°C) for usually around 48–50 hours, after which the koji can be harvested. I'll use the term koji in this book to refer to the inoculated grains: the unique building block needed to make not only miso, but also soy sauce, rice vinegar and rice wine, to name a few. I am not going to explore how to make koji at home in this book—although this is what many koji enthusiasts do—but luckily koji in its dried form is easily accessible online and in specialist Japanese stores.

- **Salt:** sea or kosher salt are my preferred options. Try to avoid salt that contains iodine or anti-caking agents. Salt allows for a safe long-term ferment at room temperature; the salt percentage when making miso or koji ferments can range from 5% to 15% or more of the total weight of soybeans and koji and is dictated by what you're making.

- **Time:** ranging from a few weeks to years, depending on the proportions of the above, your end goal (do you want a sweeter or saltier miso?) and, ultimately, your patience.

Based on your end objective, such as white miso or red miso, these elements shift: White miso is sweeter and requires less salt, more koji, and less time; red miso requires more salt, less koji, and more time. I'll go into the process for miso making in the following section; however, once the three ingredients are combined in your long-term fermentation container, the fermentation starts. The enzymes in the koji will start to digest the carbohydrates and proteins until the miso is matured to your satisfaction.

Just as wine gains complexity as it matures and ages, every batch of miso will have some variance and even once your miso is "done" you may want to continue fermenting it at room temperature to further develop the taste. View it as ever-evolving and remember that you are the judge for when it's done. And it's with this attitude toward miso, one of agency and determination, that I believe you can fully access its potential as a flavor, ingredient, and lens to view how you cook at home.

I am an advocate for learning and honoring ancient preservation traditions, but just as our ancestors adapted these techniques to what was accessible to them, I want you to view these methods as a point of departure based on your own creativity, accessibility, and locality. What if we replace soybeans with other beans? Or replace them with entirely new ingredients? I'm no purist, as my own understanding and world view derives from a confluence of cultures and adaptability as a means of survival and creativity.

There are debates within the fermentation community about what constitutes a miso; those that depart from the traditional ingredients are sometimes termed an "amino paste" or a miso-like paste. I don't lose much sleep over this debate—who can truly gate-keep a name? Do I have more authority as a person of Japanese ancestry? I don't think so, but even with my weirdest miso projects (such as miso made from chocolate cake or rehydrated dried mango), the process is based on miso. If it's a miso in terms of process and applications, and inspired by that origin, is it not also a miso?

Nowadays, miso is one of the trendiest ingredients. It is no longer reserved for Japanese cuisine and is used in endless recipes—from adding a well-balanced saltiness to desserts, to acting as a savory, umami background and adding instant flavor, especially to plant-based dishes. Yet despite becoming increasingly ubiquitous, I'd argue we've only scratched the surface of this complex and versatile ingredient. Making miso at home is an education, not just in how flavors evolve and can be harnessed, but also in pushing your own boundaries in the home kitchen.

MISO 101

View miso as a spectrum of salt, umami, and sweetness.

We've been conditioned—due to commercial availability—to view miso through a binary lens of dark versus light (or more accurately, red versus white). These two types, while ubiquitous, are a direct reflection of the proportions of soybeans, koji, and salt in those two miso varieties, as well as the amount of time needed for fermentation.

In Japan, there are countless types of miso: not just in terms of ingredients used, but also in texture and color, many of which reflect the regions in which they originated. But perhaps even more exciting (and accessible, unless you go to Japan often) are the modern twists challenging conventional assumptions about miso that are appearing across the globe—from high-end restaurants to humble home kitchens. And it's through this discourse and confluence of ideas that some of the coolest fermentation innovation is erupting.

As you embark on this journey, I want to emphasize that miso making is a rather forgiving process. This may surprise you with what may seem like an involved and complex ferment, but the actual steps are rather simple. Salt percentages and ingredient proportions follow the same general formulas. The main differentiator is dictated by the end objective: a saltier (longer) or sweeter (shorter) ferment. The eagle-eyed among you will also note that there's additional salt used throughout the miso-making process, separate from what's required as a percentage of the koji and soybeans. This additional salt is primarily used to optimize the miso's success from a safety standpoint, but is a nominal amount in relation to the total percentage of salt used so will not have a massive impact on your final product. These ranges and variables may be concerning to see in a cookbook, but I must reassure you that miso making has a lot of room for error and the finished product is truly defined by you and your taste preferences.

In this section, I'll go into the basic proportions, method, and troubleshooting for making white and red miso, followed by some of my frequently made creative spins on these traditional approaches. Note that these recipes are ultimately all about proportions and percentages, so once you get comfortable with the process, they can easily be scaled up or down if needed.

PREPARATION

—When making miso with dried legumes, I assume they will approximately double in volume when soaked and cooked. If you'd like to be more accurate with your measurements, my suggestion would be to first soak and cook your beans and then measure out the necessary proportions.

—You can use unpasteurized or homemade miso to kickstart your next batch by mixing in a few tablespoons alongside your koji and beans. I do not find this absolutely necessary, but a surge of good microbes from your existing miso can only help if you have it on hand.

—All the recipes in this section were developed using freshly made rice koji. Most commercially available koji is dehydrated (which works very well in the absence of fresh koji and is often sold in its matted form). For this reason, dehydrated koji can definitely be swapped in, but be sure to break up the dried koji so that each grain is separated. Some sources will advise you to rehydrate your dehydrated koji; however, for most miso and miso-like pastes—and those I've included here—there's usually sufficient moisture coming from the other ingredients, so there should be no need to rehydrate prior to using.

—When putting miso into your chosen container, you may struggle with removing all the air pockets, especially when making more traditional legume-based miso varieties, which tend to be denser. Using a glass jar helps here so you can quickly identify the air pockets visually. Use your hands to compact the miso; the handle of a long wooden spoon (or a pickle packer) can also help do this. Do not fret if some small visible air pockets remain as they should fill with tamari as the miso ferments, but try your best.

—Fermentation weights are key to making consistent miso and miso-like pastes as they minimize air pockets and force tamari, a by-product of making miso and a delicious umami-packed sauce in itself, to gather on the miso's surface, which then helps preserve it safely as it ferments. Most resources suggest using a weight that is equal to the weight of the miso. In my experience, I'm usually limited by the size of the jar so I just do my best to add as much weight as possible. Some weight is better than no weight! My preferred fermentation weight is actually quite simple (and resourceful!): I fill a food-safe plastic bag with dried rice or legumes, or even salt. Plastic bags work well since you can spread the bottom of the bag to cover the entire surface of the miso, which then limits its exposure to oxygen. I would not advise filling food-safe plastic bags with liquid as these can easily leak and ruin your ferment.

DURING FERMENTATION

—Check your miso regularly. During the initial fermentation period, as the salt draws out liquid, tamari should start to pool at the top of your miso, a very positive sign. The tamari also acts as a barrier to oxygen (remember, "everything is fine below the brine!"). If you have a lot of tamari, you can harvest some of it and use it as you'd use a soy sauce (albeit more delicate in taste in my opinion), but the best practice is to leave it with your miso.

—Keep an eye out for any yeast or mold growth, particularly on the surface where the miso is exposed to oxygen. If you notice this—at any point during its fermentation life cycle—simply scrape it off, sprinkle a small amount of salt on the surface, and reposition the fermentation weight.

POST-FERMENTATION

—Homemade miso will always continue to ferment, as it's not pasteurized. As with other ferments in this book, move it to the fridge when you're happy with its flavor (and if you're not, continue to ferment it). There is no need to keep the fermentation weight on the miso once it's in the fridge. I like to divide a batch at this point, keeping one container in the fridge and the rest at room temperature to observe how the flavor evolves.

—Decanting miso may seem a bit intimidating but is quite straightforward: Carefully remove the weight, wipe down the sides of the container with a clean towel, and remove the top layer of the miso if there's any mold or yeast. It may be discolored or a bit too funky, but all of the miso underneath that top layer, which may have been exposed to oxygen, is safe for consumption.

—If your miso is covered by a layer of tamari, you can either harvest the tamari as a separate ingredient or mix it into your miso.

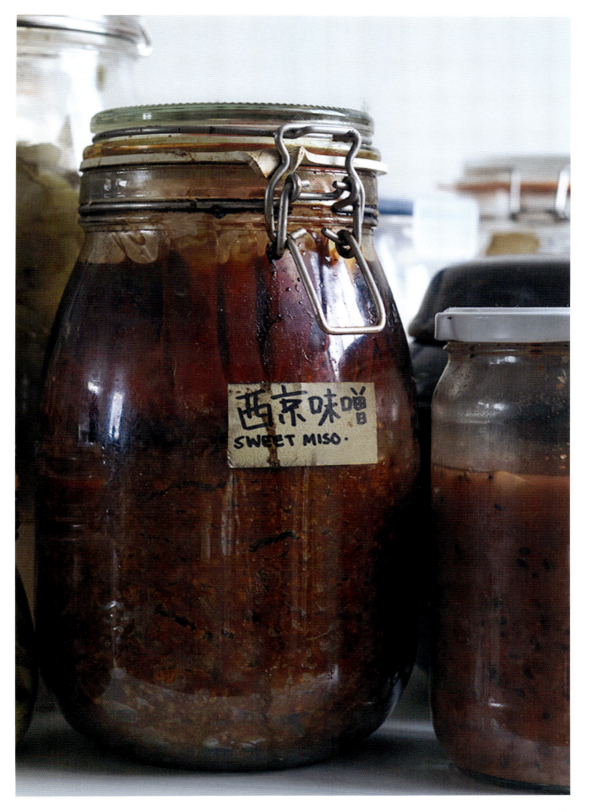

WHITE MISO AND RED MISO

The process of making white and red miso is very similar, with only slight variations in the proportions of ingredients and the time needed for fermentation.

White miso is sweeter and relatively mild in taste, hence is often used with more delicate ingredients, such as fish or desserts. It is fermented for a short period of time (as quick as a few weeks and up to 3 months), and consequently doesn't require too much salt (in the range of 6–8%). It also requires a higher proportion of koji to soybeans than red miso (approximately equal parts cooked soybeans to koji).

Red miso is darker and more robust in flavor, and is what I use most in my cooking due to its versatility. Yes, it is saltier, but that just means I may use a bit less if a dish requires a less salty or lighter miso. Red miso requires a higher proportion of soybeans to koji (2:1 parts cooked soybeans to koji) and as it's a longer-term ferment, requires more salt (12–15%). I tend to start checking my red miso after 6 months, but it can continue to ferment indefinitely.

I make miso throughout the year but traditionally, and this is true of many longer-term ferments, miso making starts during the colder winter months to allow for a slower fermentation, which results in a more nuanced and complex flavor. With all miso varieties, the traditional soybean can be swapped with other legumes—my favorites in my home kitchen being chickpeas, split peas, and black and kidney beans. Regardless of what you use, I strongly suggest cooking them from their dried form. It is a longer process with the soaking and cooking; this just means that making miso with dried beans can take place over several days, which is very short given how much time is needed for the subsequent fermentation, so sit tight! *See step-by-step images on pages 92–93.*

PREP TIME: 30–45 MINUTES + 12–18 hours soaking
COOK TIME: 20 MINUTES–4 HOURS depending on method
FERMENTATION TIME: 2 WEEKS–3 MONTHS (white), 6+ MONTHS (red)

Basic recipe continues on the next page

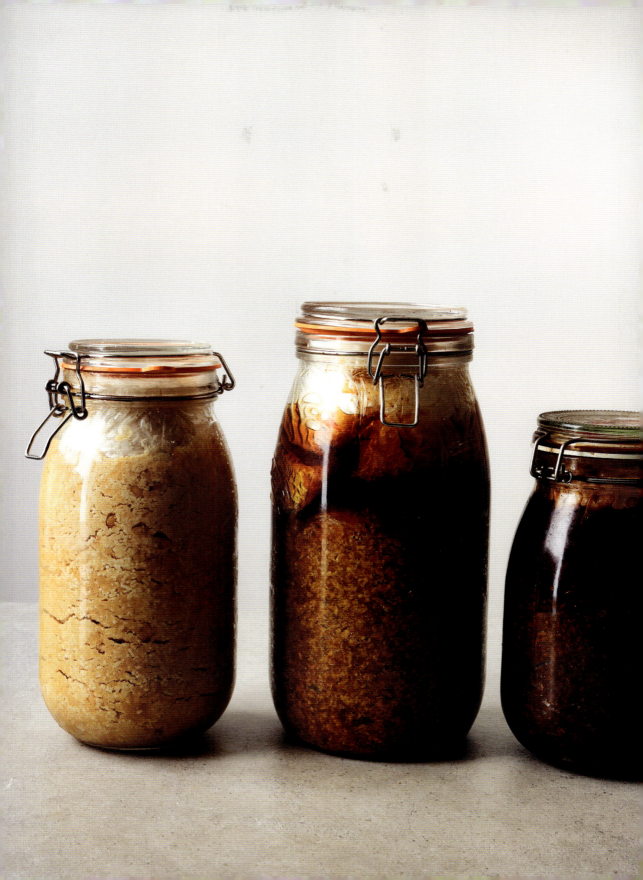

This makes approximately 1kg (2.25lbs) of miso; you will need a jar that is one-and-a-half to two times that size to allow room for a fermentation weight

FOR WHITE MISO (1:1 PARTS COOKED SOYBEANS TO KOJI)

250g (9oz) dried soybeans

500g (1lb 2oz) koji

salt (8% of the total weight of the cooked soybeans and koji)

1 tbsp unpasteurized miso (optional)

FOR RED MISO (2:1 PARTS COOKED SOYBEANS TO KOJI)

300g (10.5oz) dried soybeans

300g (10.5oz) koji

salt (13% of the total weight of the cooked soybeans and koji)

1 tbsp unpasteurized miso (optional)

SPECIAL EQUIPMENT: food processor (optional)

In a large bowl, rinse and soak the dried soybeans in fresh water for 12–18 hours, ensuring they are fully submerged and topping up with fresh water as needed. After they're sufficiently soaked, rinse and drain them.

Cook the soybeans in water until they are soft and easily crushable between your fingers. The exact cooking time depends on the method of cooking: from 20–25 minutes in a pressure cooker to 3–4 hours on the stove. If cooking them on the stove, keep an eye on the water, as it may need a top-up as it boils.

Drain the cooked soybeans, reserving 240ml (1 cup) of the cooking liquid, which you may need to add to the miso mixture to attain the correct consistency.

In a very large bowl (large enough to hold the soybeans and koji), and while the soybeans are still warm, mash them to your desired consistency: I tend to use my hands, squeezing the soybeans into a chunky texture, but sometimes opt for a food processor, which creates a smoother miso (and is much faster). I prefer chunkier miso—the ingredients will continue to break down as they ferment and you can always purée it further if needed. Add a very small amount (1 tablespoon at a time) of the cooking liquid if needed; however, I rarely add liquid if the soybeans are thoroughly cooked.

The mashed soybeans should be at room temperature at this point: If they are still hot, wait until they're at room temperature before adding the final ingredients as very hot temperatures can inhibit the activity of the koji.

Add the koji, salt, and unpasteurized miso (if using). Using your hands, knead everything together thoroughly to ensure the koji and salt are evenly distributed throughout the mashed soybeans. If using dried koji, you may need to add additional cooking liquid to loosen the mixture—you're aiming for a dough-like texture that isn't too wet.

Use your hands to form balls (ping-pong ball size) of the mixture; if you're scaling the recipe up, the size can be increased to a tennis ball size. Use force to ensure they're free of air pockets.

Prepare your fermentation container by pouring in 1 tablespoon of the cooking liquid and giving the container a shake so that the interior is lightly coated in liquid. Dump out any residual liquid and sprinkle 1 tablespoon of salt inside the container so that the bottom and sides are covered with a light coating of salt. Do not stress if this is not perfect: It acts only as an additional safety net for preservation.

Now fill your container with the balls of miso. This is a traditional method to ensure air pockets are minimized and the miso is really packed in with force. Put the balls in your container in a single layer and then mash them down with your fist. Be diligent in making sure there are no obvious pockets of air and continue to press down with force with each new layer. You can use your hands, a pickle packer, or a wooden spoon.

Continue this process until you've filled your jar with miso. Flatten the top layer with your hands and sprinkle with 1 teaspoon of salt. The miso should be dry enough that you're essentially dusting the top layer with salt and it shouldn't immediately absorb into the miso.

To limit exposure to oxygen, place a layer of parchment paper or plastic wrap over the entire top layer of miso, ensuring that it fits as well as possible. Wipe the sides of the container clean to remove any residual miso mixture that could attract unwanted mold.

Add a fermentation weight on top of the miso; this may be limited by the size of the container, but aim for a weight that is as close as possible to the weight of the miso. I like to fill a food-safe plastic bag with dried rice, beans, or salt, which allows consistent coverage across the top layer of miso. Put the lid on the container and let the fermentation commence!

Leave the miso in a cool place out of direct sunlight and ferment for a minimum of 2 weeks and up to 3 months for a white or lighter miso or 6 months or more for a red or darker miso. When you're happy with the flavor, move it to the fridge, which will slow down the fermentation process; otherwise continue fermenting it until it's reached your desired taste.

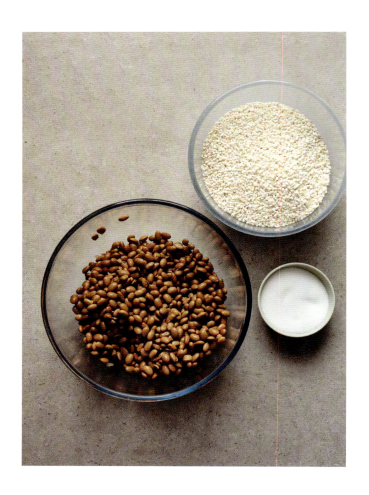
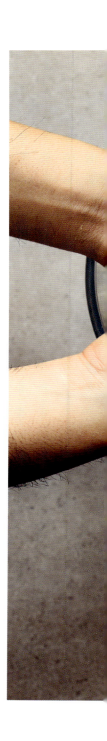

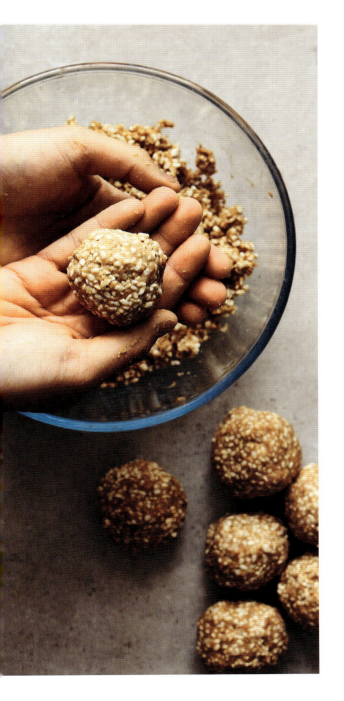
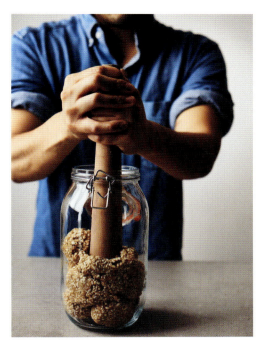

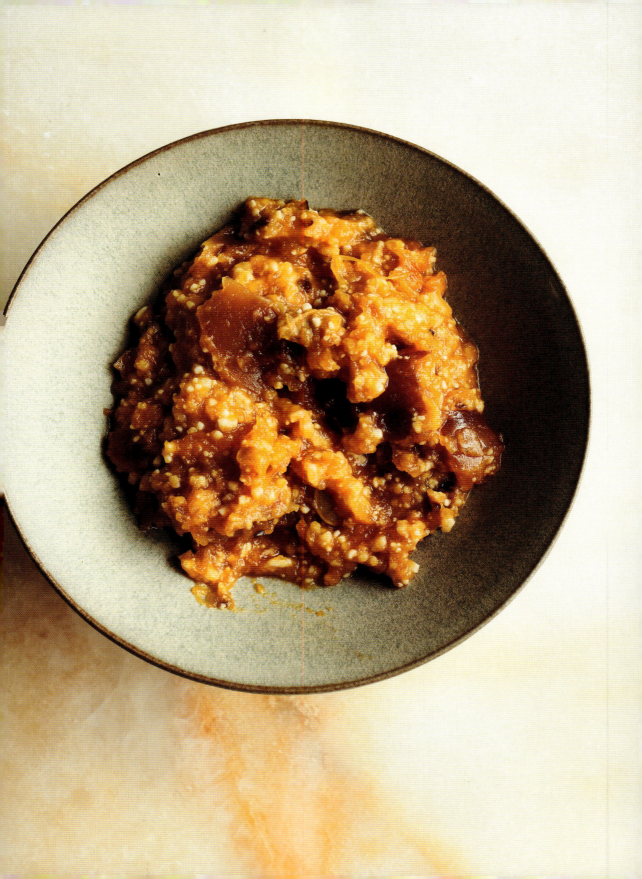

PUMPKIN MISO

Memories of food are some of my deepest: my grandmother pan-frying chicken with chopsticks, with such deft choreography despite her arthritic hands; sitting around our kitchen table making triangular rice balls, filled with sour pickled plum or savory seaweed; winters in Chicago, steaming kabocha pumpkin in miso soup, the miso spiralling as I dipped chopsticks into the comforting warmth. And therein lies the inspiration for pumpkin miso.

Is this actually a miso? Good question. In the truest definition, no, as it's missing the vital ingredient of soybeans. However, in terms of process, end product, and applications it is similar to miso, packed with umami but intense with natural pumpkin sweetness. Not all pumpkins are created equal: Use ones with less water content (I generally avoid seasonal Halloween pumpkins), or cut the pumpkin into smaller pieces before roasting.

In terms of applications, this miso can be used as you'd use any other type of miso, but it obviously tastes intensely pumpkin-like, which I think lends itself particularly well to soups (such as my Green Mean Bean Miso Soup on page 198) and sweets (such as my Miso Tahini Chocolate Chip Blondies on page 239).

PREP TIME: 20–30 MINUTES | COOK TIME: 40–60 MINUTES
FERMENTATION TIME: 6+ MONTHS

This makes approximately 1kg (2.25lbs) of miso; you will need a jar that is one-and-a-half to two times that size to allow room for a fermentation weight

650g (1lb 7oz) pumpkin
1–2 tsp vegetable oil
325g (11.5oz) koji
salt (13% of the total weight of the cooked pumpkin and koji)

SPECIAL EQUIPMENT: food processor (optional)

Preheat the oven to 425°F (220°C).

Cut your pumpkin into large pieces (approximately 5cm/2in cubes)—no need to discard the skin and seeds. Cutting the pumpkin into chunks will increase its surface area and reduce moisture content.

Coat the pumpkin pieces lightly in oil and bake on a baking sheet for 40–60 minutes, until nicely caramelized and fork tender.

If you want to be precise, weigh the roasted pumpkin and measure out 50% of that weight in koji. For example, if the weight of the roasted pumpkin is 625g (1lb 6oz), measure out 313g (11oz) of koji.

Recipe continues on the next page

Combine the pumpkin and koji and measure out 13% of the combined weight in salt (13% of 938g/2lbs = 122g/4.5oz of salt).

Using a food processor (or your hands), mash the cooked pumpkin, koji, and salt together until fully incorporated. Do not worry if there are still chunks of seed or koji as they'll break down as the miso ferments. This mixture will most likely be more moist than legume-based miso varieties, and for that reason, I do not add any additional salt to the interior of the jar.

Fill your container with the pumpkin miso. Look out for any large pockets of air and aim to remove these by pressing down with a spoon or by shaking the jar with force—oxygen is not your friend when making miso.

Flatten the top layer and sprinkle with 1 teaspoon of salt, followed by a piece of parchment paper or plastic wrap, ensuring that it fits as well as possible over the entire top layer of miso. Wipe the sides of the container clean to remove any residual miso mixture that could attract unwanted mold.

Add a fermentation weight on top of the miso; this may be limited by the size of the container, but aim for a weight that is as close as possible to the weight of the miso. I like to fill a food-safe plastic bag with dried rice, beans, or salt, which allows consistent coverage across the top layer of miso. Put the lid on the container and let the fermentation commence!

Leave the jar in a cool place out of direct sunlight and ferment for a minimum of 6 months and up to a year. Start tasting it after 6 months.

When you're happy with the flavor, move it to the fridge, which will slow down the fermentation process; otherwise continue fermenting it until it's reached your desired taste.

GARLIC MISOZUKE

Did you know that you can use miso as a pickling bed? Misozuke, or "pickled in miso," is one of my favorite tsukemono (Japanese pickles) varieties and this garlic version is as simple as it can get, but punches hard with flavor. As the garlic ferments and matures in the miso, the cloves absorb all of the flavor from the miso, producing a deeply sweet and savory garlic pickle.

Eat the cloves whole, or slice them thinly to add to a pickle platter or atop crackers with a soft cheese. Chopping them finely for the base of a dish is a great way to build flavor, but you may soon find out that you need to ration your miso-pickled garlic as it goes quickly! The best thing about this pickle is that you end up with two delicious products: the miso-pickled garlic and garlic-flavored miso.

This method of pickling works particularly well with denser vegetables such as daikon radish (mooli), carrot, and celery. However, if you experiment with other vegetables, check them regularly as they'll emit water as they ferment.

PREP TIME: 15 MINUTES | FERMENTATION TIME: 2-3 MONTHS minimum

Makes 10-12 fermented cloves

- 200g (7oz) red or dark miso (if using store-bought, ensure it's unpasteurized)
- 1 head of garlic, cloves separated and peeled, root ends sliced off

Add a layer of miso to a jar followed by a single layer of garlic cloves. Use a clean spoon to push each layer down firmly to minimize any air pockets. Repeat this process until you've used all the garlic, ensuring that the final layer of garlic cloves is entirely covered in miso.

Leave the jar in a cool place out of direct sunlight and ferment at room temperature indefinitely. As long as the garlic is covered in a layer of miso, it should stay safe and not lead to any blooms of yeast or mold. I think the garlic is best after 2-3 months. Once you're happy with the flavor, move it to the fridge to slow down fermentation; otherwise continue fermenting it until it's reached your desired taste.

Before eating or using in your home cooking, you can either wipe the miso away from the garlic or simply keep the residual miso for additional flavor.

BEET MISO WITH CUMIN & ALLSPICE

This recipe is conceptually similar to the pumpkin miso in that it's using a vegetable instead of beans and is entirely zero-waste, using the whole beet, skin and all—with two distinct differences: It's a faster ferment with less salt and more koji (in other words, it follows the white miso method), which results in a sweeter and "fresher" paste, and most interestingly, it includes spices.

The additional spices make this "miso" slightly unconventional and perhaps less versatile, but as someone who loves beet in all forms, I encourage you to try it. It's earthy, sweet, and ultimately quite complex due to the spices, which really complement the beet. Delicious in a borscht, dal, or even as the base for a beet-cured salmon. *See the photo on the next page.*

PREP TIME: 20–30 MINUTES | COOK TIME: 40–60 MINUTES
FERMENTATION TIME: 3 MONTHS

This makes approximately 1kg (2.25lbs) of miso; you will need a jar that is one-and-a-half to two times that size to allow room for a fermentation weight

- **500g (1lb 2oz) whole beets**
- **1–2 tsp vegetable oil**
- **500g (1lb 2oz) koji**
- **salt (5% of the total weight of the cooked beet and koji)**
- **1 tsp freshly ground cumin seeds**
- **1 tsp freshly ground allspice**

SPECIAL EQUIPMENT: food processor

Preheat the oven to 425°F (220°C).

Wash and dry the beets. Coat the whole beets lightly in oil and bake on a baking sheet for 40–60 minutes until fork tender.

Leave the beets to cool for 10–15 minutes before starting the next step.

If you want to be precise, weigh the roasted beet and measure out the same weight in koji. For example, if the cooked beet weighs 450g (1lb), measure out 450g (1lb) of koji. Combine the beet and koji and measure out 5% of the combined weight in salt (5% of 900g/2lbs = 45g/1.5oz of salt).

Using a food processor, blend the roasted beet, koji, salt, and ground spices together (if the beets are particularly large, cut them into smaller pieces before blending). This mixture will most likely be more moist than legume-based miso varieties, and for that reason, I do not add any additional salt to the interior of the jar.

Fill your container with the beet miso. Look out for any large pockets of air and aim to remove these by pressing down with a spoon or by shaking the jar with force—oxygen is not your friend when making miso.

Flatten the top layer and sprinkle with 1 teaspoon of salt, followed by a piece of parchment paper or plastic wrap, ensuring that it fits as well as possible over the entire top layer of miso. Wipe the sides of the container clean to remove any residual miso mixture that could attract unwanted mold.

Add a fermentation weight on top of the miso; this may be limited by the size of the container, but aim for a weight that is as close as possible to the weight of the miso. I like to fill a food-safe plastic bag with dried rice, beans, or salt, which allows consistent coverage across the top layer of miso. Put the lid on the container and let the fermentation commence!

Leave the jar in a cool place out of direct sunlight and ferment for 2–3 months.

When you're happy with the flavor, move it to the fridge, which will slow down the fermentation process; otherwise continue fermenting it until it's reached your desired taste.

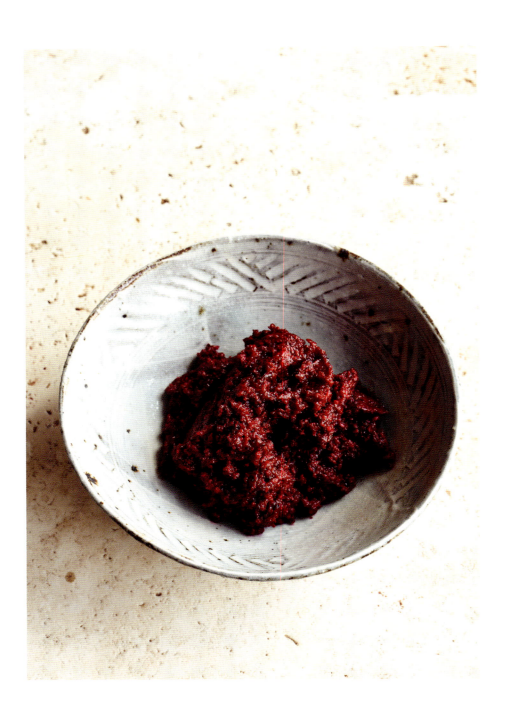

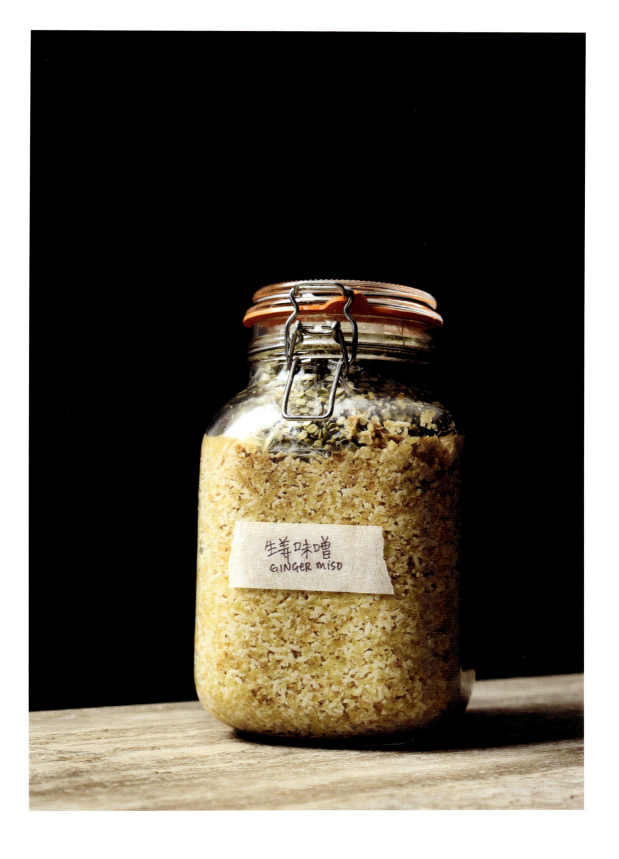

GINGER MISO

Although I endeavor to combat food waste as much as possible in my kitchen, ginger was one of the ingredients that would inevitably end up in the compost bin—either sadly desiccated if left at room temperature, or soggy and rather unpleasant from fridge neglect. This ginger "miso" is my answer to this problem—and as you may expect, it can be easily adapted based on what aromatics you have kicking about. The end result, which you can start tucking into after just a few weeks, is a sweet and intensely gingery umami paste which can (and should) be used in any savory recipe where ginger is required. You could throw a teaspoon into stir-fries, curries, marinades, and sauces.

An obvious riff on this recipe is a play on the ubiquitous ginger-garlic paste of South Asia. You can use 50:50 ginger and garlic, or throw in a few chiles for good measure, but stick with equal parts aromatics to koji.

I tend to move this ferment to the fridge after about a month, since as soon as I start using it, it can quickly oxidize (you'll usually see a slight darkening in the color). This is not harmful, but keeping it in the fridge, flattening it down after each use, and covering the top with a piece of parchment paper or plastic wrap should keep oxidation at bay. *See photo on previous page.*

PREP TIME: 20 MINUTES | FERMENTATION TIME: 2–5 WEEKS

This makes approximately 400g (14oz) of miso; you will need a jar that is one-and-a-half to two times that size to allow room for a fermentation weight

200g (7oz) fresh ginger, peeled and roughly chopped

200g (7oz) koji

salt (5% of the total weight of above ingredients)

SPECIAL EQUIPMENT: food processor

Put the ginger, koji, and salt into a food processor and blitz to a rough paste.

Fill your container with the ginger paste. Look out for any large pockets of air and aim to remove these by pressing down with a spoon or by shaking the jar with force—oxygen is not your friend when making miso.

Flatten the top and sprinkle with 1 teaspoon of salt, followed by a piece of parchment paper or plastic wrap, ensuring that it fits as well as possible over the entire top layer of miso. Wipe the sides of the container clean to remove any residual miso mixture that could attract unwanted mold.

Add a fermentation weight on top of the miso; this may be limited by the size of the container, but aim for a weight that is as close as possible to the weight of the miso. I like to fill a food-safe plastic bag with dried rice, beans, or salt, which allows consistent coverage across the top layer of miso. Put the lid on the container and let the fermentation commence!

Leave your jar in a dark and cool place for 2–5 weeks and then move to the fridge. This can be quite a liquidy miso—especially as it starts to ferment—so put a plate underneath to catch any brine. The jar may also need to be burped occasionally. Start tasting (and using) after the first 2 weeks and move to the fridge after around 5 weeks.

KOJI CHIMICHURRI PASTE

This is a really fun and vibrant recipe and an homage to many of my favorite herbaceous condiments, celebrating the complementary flavors in South America's chimichurri and Japan's kanzuri and yuzu kosho. These initial sources of inspiration have each given elements to this final product: parsley from chimichurri, koji from kanzuri, citrus from yuzu kosho, and the unifying ingredient building common ground across these traditions: chiles. As expected, this creates a bold and bright chile paste that should be used in small quantities. It is particularly good as a condiment or in a marinade for grilled meat and vegetables.

PREP TIME: 20 MINUTES | FERMENTATION TIME: 2–3 MONTHS minimum

This makes approximately 400g (14oz) of paste; you will need a jar that is one-and-a-half to two times that size to allow room for a fermentation weight

- 150g (5oz) mixed chiles (a combination of both mild and hot, based on your preference), roughly chopped
- 100g (3.5oz) grated citrus zest (a combination of lemon, lime, and orange)
- 100g (3.5oz) fresh parsley (leaves and stems), or a combination of parsley and cilantro, roughly chopped
- 175g (6oz) koji
- salt (12% of the total weight of above ingredients)

SPECIAL EQUIPMENT: food processor

Put all of the ingredients into a food processor and blitz to a paste.

Fill your container with the paste. Look out for any large pockets of air and aim to remove these by pressing down with a spoon or by shaking the jar with force—oxygen is not your friend when making koji-based ferments.

Flatten the top and sprinkle with 1 teaspoon of salt, followed by a piece of parchment paper or plastic wrap, ensuring that it fits as well as possible over the entire top layer of paste. Wipe the sides of the container clean to remove any residual mixture that could attract unwanted mold.

Add a fermentation weight on top; this may be limited by the size of the container, but aim for a weight that is as close as possible to the weight of the paste. I like to fill a food-safe plastic bag with dried rice, beans, or salt, which allows consistent coverage across the top layer. Put the lid on the container and let the fermentation commence!

Leave the jar in a cool place out of direct sunlight and ferment indefinitely. As this is more of a fermented chile paste and will be used in small amounts, you can start tasting and using it after 2–3 months; however, remember that it will be salty, especially when it's younger. When you're happy with the flavor, move it to the fridge, which will slow down the fermentation process; otherwise continue fermenting it until it's reached your desired taste.

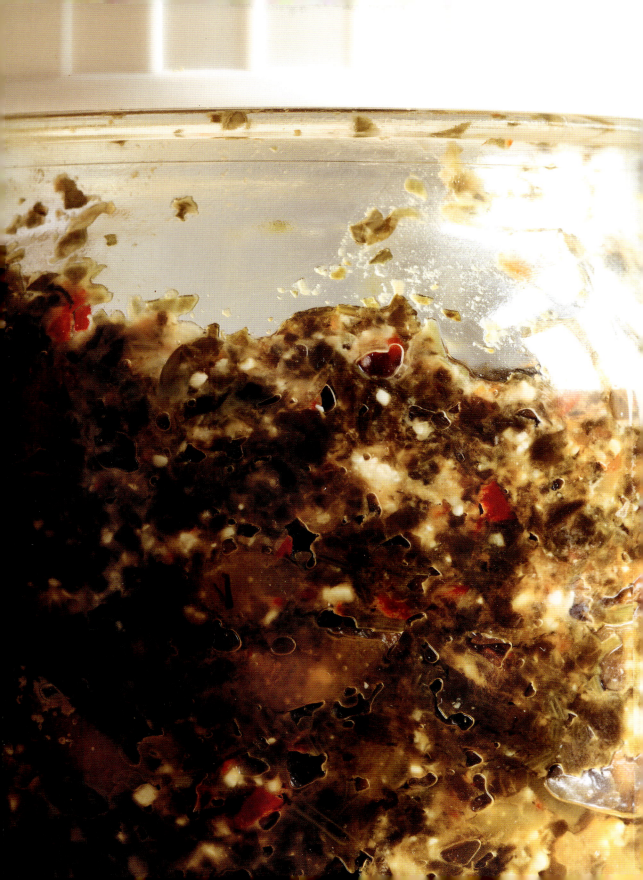

PICKLING

This book would be incomplete without what I like to call everyday pickles. Thanks to sugar and acid, usually in the form of vinegar, these pickles offer the quintessential zingy brightness most people expect from a pickle. Where fermentation brings the funk, these pickles bring a sweet and sour tang to the party. These pickles are likely familiar to you: sweet cucumber slices atop burgers, shredded daikon radish (mooli) and carrot in Southeast Asian cuisine, or the ubiquitous quick-pickled red onion, which immediately adds intrigue to whatever you're eating with its ruby color.

I grew up in Chicago, a liberal urban bubble in a part of the USA abundant with farmland. Visiting our local farmers market was a weekly event for my family every Saturday morning. At what sometimes felt like an ungodly hour, my sister and I jumped into the back of my dad's station wagon, my mom with reusable cloth bags in hand (as well as baked goods for her farmer friends). I was always half-asleep, and the comfort of family and routine would often lull me to sleep during that ten-minute drive: Simon and Garfunkel playing from the radio, the distinct smell of sun concentrated against the car. And like clockwork, as soon as I'd fallen asleep, we were there.

For the next hour, we'd walk from stall to stall, my parents catching up with the farmers they bought from weekly, me running off to sample whatever freebies were available that day, all against a backdrop of color and flavor: a seasonal mosaic of gladioli and gourds, brassicas and corn. I've now come to realize just how formative this family ritual was: not just a lesson in seasonality, nor on the importance of supporting farmers directly, but through what I tasted and the indelible mark it left on my sense memories. We would routinely visit our family's favorite seller, a farmer from Michigan who stood apart from the rest with their jars of preserved goods. I relished (no pun intended) their sweet pickles, spiced with complex aromatics, and constantly changing to reflect their surplus produce. As I exchanged pleasantries and small talk with the farmers—many of whom had seen me grow up over the years—my eyes darted across their seasonal offerings with complete enchantment. *What new flavors could illuminate our taste buds? Which produce has been preserved at its prime? And how could this all be combined to create something truly beautiful?* Perhaps I was subconsciously planning future pickle platter ideas and flavor combinations, but as a child this sensory overload of sights and flavors left me wanting to further explore this epicurean desire.

PICKLES 101

The method of pickling in this section is notably different from the fermentation methods outlined earlier. Both require an acidic environment for shelf-stable preservation, but in this case, the pickling relies on immersing vegetables and fruits in an acidic brine. I am a massive fan of raw apple cider vinegar (i.e., one with live cultures) and use this for nearly all of my pickles that require vinegar. I love the fruitiness it adds, which complements all pickles, and as it is unpasteurized, it also adds some healthy bacteria. Plain distilled white vinegar can be used as an alternative due to its neutral taste. Red or white wine vinegar can also work but will impact the flavor—and hue, in the case of the former—of the final pickle.

The vinegar, water, sugar, and salt ratios can vary according to what you're trying to create, as well as personal taste. Depending on who you ask (or what you read), there are many "golden rules" for proportions: A common one is to use equal parts vinegar to water and then season to taste. One of my favorites (and very easy to remember) is 3:2:1, referring to three parts vinegar to two parts water to one part sugar. (This is easy if you measure them by volume.) Both of these rules can be changed according to your taste—perhaps more acidity from vinegar or additional sugar, if needed. That said, these proportions generally refer to the necessary vinegar content for longer-term storage, and the focus in this section is on fridge-friendly pickles and quick pickles, recipes meant to be eaten relatively quickly and kept in the fridge for when you're in need of a sweet pickle hit.

A few notes:

—Technically all of these pickles can last indefinitely in the fridge. However, texturally, the pickles will change as water is drawn out from the vegetables, so try these often to determine what you like best!

—As sugar is used in these pickle recipes primarily for flavor, the amount and type can be changed to your personal taste. Sugar alternatives include honey, maple syrup, and agave.

—Not surprisingly, I like to reuse my vinegar-based brine—not just for pickles, for which I generally reuse it only once, but also as an ingredient for sauces, dressings, and whenever acidity and sweetness are needed in a dish. However, taste it before you commit to its second usage. Pickle brines will become diluted over time depending on the water content of the vegetables being pickled, so if it tastes sour enough, use it for a second batch of pickles, otherwise repurpose it as an ingredient.

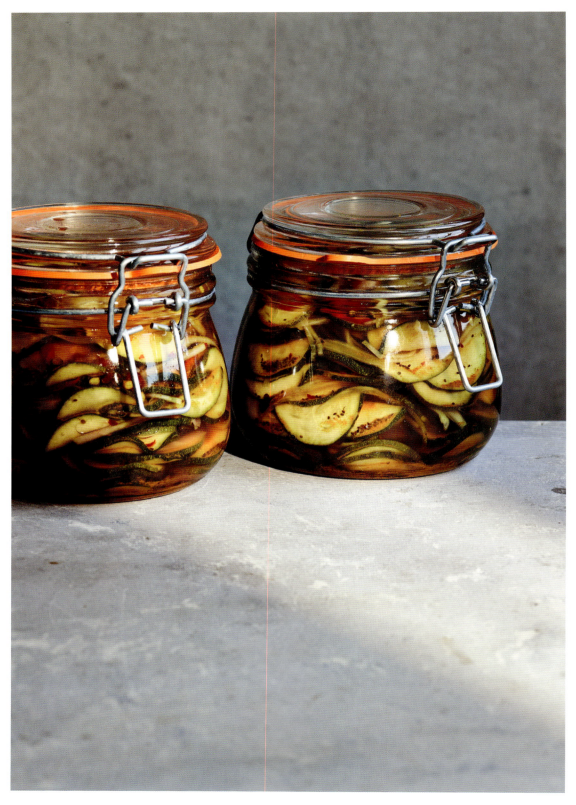

ZUCCHINI BREAD & BUTTER PICKLES

This is what I call an all-purpose pickle. The flavors should be familiar—sweet and salty, fruity and acidic—and for me, it takes me back to my childhood. It reminds me of my local farmers market in Chicago, running off ahead of my mom to grab a sample of these pickles, a satisfying burst of flavor and a respite from those hot summer days. It's particularly good between bread (hence the name?): in summer barbecue burgers or tuna sandwiches (or the Sweet Pickle Tuna Summer Rolls on page 205). This recipe is versatile both in quantity and variety—and, case in point, I've swapped the traditional cucumber with zucchini. If you can find pickling cucumbers, use those, but zucchini (and similar-size summer squash) is more accessible to me and better mimics the texture of denser cucumbers.

PREP TIME: 20 MINUTES + 2 hours salting
PICKLING TIME: 24 HOURS plus chilling

Makes two 500-ml (1-pint) jars

- 500g (1lb 2oz) zucchini, cut into 5-mm (¼-in) rounds
- 1 red onion, peeled, cut in half, and thinly sliced
- 1 mild chile, thinly sliced, deseeded
- 1 tbsp salt
- 500ml (2 cups plus 1 tbsp) apple cider vinegar
- 200g (7oz) sugar
- 1 tsp ground turmeric
- 1 tsp red pepper flakes
- 1 tsp yellow mustard seeds
- 1 tsp coriander seeds
- 1 tsp celery seeds

Put the thinly sliced vegetables into a large bowl, add the salt, and mix thoroughly. Leave for 2 hours, stirring every 30 minutes or so (or when you remember). You should notice water gathering at the bottom of the bowl.

While the vegetables are salting, make the brine. In a small saucepan, gently warm the apple cider vinegar and sugar together, along with all of the spices. Once the sugar has dissolved, remove the pan from the heat and leave the brine to infuse with flavor until it is lukewarm.

While the brine cools, gently squeeze the salted zucchini, onion, and chile, reserving the liquid, and divide them evenly between two clean jars.

Add the brine squeezed from the vegetables to the vinegar brine. Top up the jars with this brine and leave them at room temperature for 24 hours before moving them to the fridge.

The pickles will be ready to eat within 24 hours but are best after 3–4 days. They will keep indefinitely.

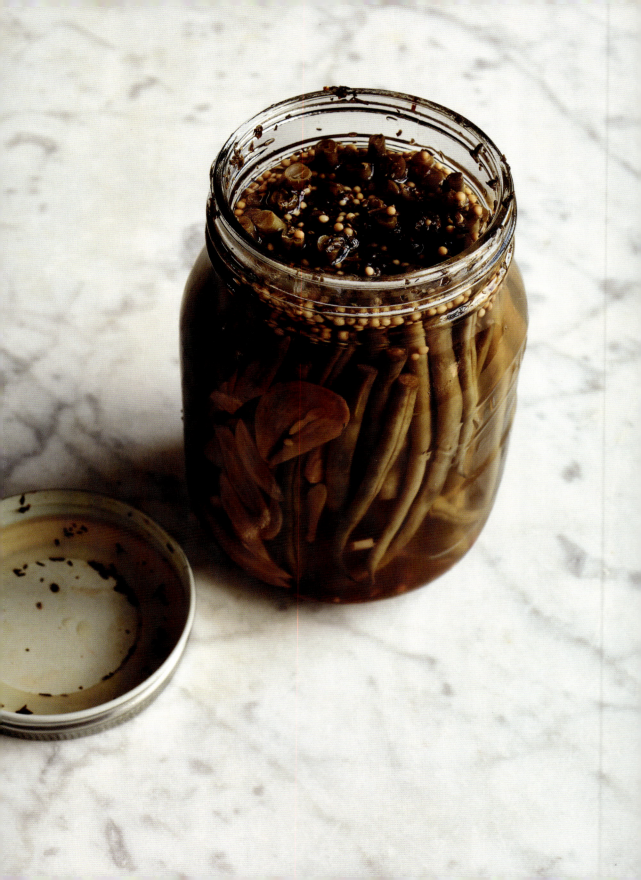

SPICY GREEN BEANS

This was one of my favorite jarred pickles from my local farmers market in Chicago. It was one of the few "spicier" pickles my parents bought, which was something quite exciting as a child, as both of my parents have low tolerances for chile heat. As with all pickles, you can adjust the spice to your liking: I've layered heat with both dried and fresh chiles—you can use fruitier chile varieties such as gochugaru or Aleppo pepper.

These are great munching pickles and generally maintain their crunch, so they can be quite hard to put down. If you're looking for something fun to do with them, chop them up for a pickled bean relish, which would be excellent with sausages at your next barbecue.

PREP TIME: 30 MINUTES | PICKLING TIME: 24 HOURS plus chilling

Makes one 500-ml (1-pint) jar

- 200g (7oz) green beans
- 2 garlic cloves, peeled and thinly sliced
- 1 mild chile, thinly sliced, deseeded if preferred
- 50g (1.75oz) sugar
- 180ml (¾ cup) apple cider vinegar
- 1½ tsp salt
- ½ tsp red pepper flakes
- 1 tsp dried thyme
- 1 tsp yellow mustard seeds

Prepare the green beans: Remove their tops and aim to trim them so they fit the full length of your jar; cutting them in half will also work but try to cut them to similar lengths.

To pack the jar: Start with the garlic and fresh chile, followed by the green beans.

To make the brine, put the sugar, apple cider vinegar, salt, and 120ml (½ cup) water into a small saucepan.

Add the aromatics. Put the pan over a low heat until the liquid reaches a gentle simmer. Immediately remove from the heat and let the sugar dissolve and aromatics infuse the brine.

When the brine has cooled slightly (it doesn't need to be room temperature), pour it over the green beans, ensuring that the brine completely covers them.

If there's any extra brine that doesn't fit into your jar, keep it for a new pickle.

Keep the jar at room temperature for 24 hours and then move it to the fridge. The pickles are best enjoyed after 3–5 days. They will keep indefinitely.

QUICK-PICKLED KOMBUCHA CHILES

These pickled chiles are not only a great way to minimize food waste (of which single chiles are prime victims!), but are one of the easiest ways to embellish a meal with heat and tang. Keep a jar of these on hand in your fridge.

These are slightly more than "quick," as I find them best after a full day of pickling, but you can of course dig in sooner if needed! Vinegar can be used here but I've found kombucha to work really well. As the acidity is generally lower than commercially available vinegar, this pickle should be kept in the fridge. No additional water is needed to allow the acid to work quickly.

This pickle is easily adaptable. You can scale it down if you want to use fewer chiles, but follow the same proportions for the brine: 3 parts kombucha (or vinegar) to 1 part sugar. I like to keep it simple, using a variety of fresh chiles, but you can throw in thinly sliced garlic, ginger, or other aromatic combinations (½ teaspoon each of coriander seeds, mustard seeds, and fennel seeds work beautifully).

PREP TIME: 15 MINUTES | PICKLING TIME: 24 HOURS plus chilling

Makes one 500-ml (1-pint) jar

- 300–400g (10.5–14oz) mixed chiles (mild, spicy, you decide)
- 50g (1.75oz) sugar
- 180ml (¾ cup) kombucha (alternatively use vinegar)
- 1½ tsp salt

Prepare your chiles: I tend to slice them thinly if using medium-size chiles; if using smaller, hotter varieties, such as bird's eye chiles, you may want to keep them whole, as chopping them up will make the brine and the finished pickled chiles much spicier.

Pack your jar with the chiles.

To make the brine, put the sugar, kombucha, and salt into a small saucepan over a low heat until it reaches a gentle simmer. Immediately remove from the heat and let the sugar dissolve.

When the brine has cooled slightly (it doesn't need to be room temperature), pour it over the chiles, ensuring the brine completely covers them.

If there's any extra brine that doesn't fit into your jar, keep it for a new pickle.

Keep the jar at room temperature for 24 hours and then move it to the fridge. The pickles are best enjoyed after 2–3 days, but if you're in a pinch, they can be eaten after 24 hours. They will keep indefinitely.

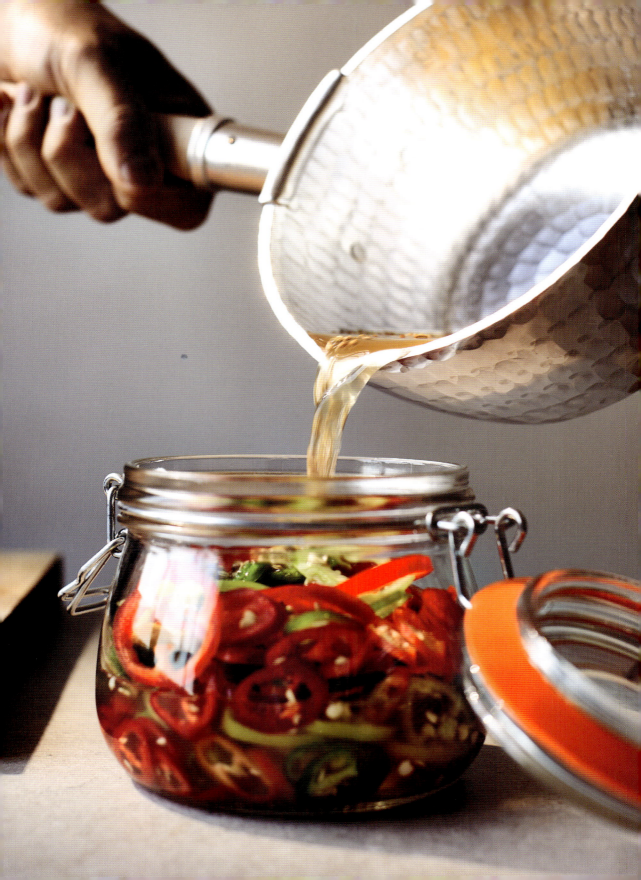

QUICK-PICKLED RED ONIONS

This recipe is very simple and is the best answer for when you need a bright acidic fix but have limited time. Once you've made this a few times, I'm confident you'll commit it to memory!

With such a simple pickle, there are many variations in flavor to explore. I like to stick with citrus as the main flavor, as it's neutrally bright enough to go with any dish. That said, you can add other aromatics or spices, with a few of my favorites being:

— ½ tsp coriander or fennel seeds, red pepper flakes, black peppercorns, sumac, whole star anise
— a few sliced garlic cloves, fresh chile, or thin slices of orange
— fresh or dried bay leaf, thyme, mint, basil

Red onions turn a vivid pink color, but you can use white or brown onions or shallots (or try a combination of several types of onions, including red). You can scale this down if you want to use just one onion, but follow the same proportions for the brine: 3 parts vinegar to 1 part sugar. These quick pickles don't need water in the brine, allowing the vinegar's acidity to work quickly.

PREP TIME: 15 MINUTES | PICKLING TIME: 1–24 HOURS

Makes one 500-ml (1-pint) jar

300–400g (10.5–14oz) red onions, peeled
1 lemon
50g (1.75oz) sugar
180ml (¾ cup) apple cider vinegar
1½ tsp salt

Prepare the red onions by slicing them thinly: The thinner you cut them, the faster they'll pickle.

Peel two strips of lemon rind and remove any pith, which will be bitter; alternatively you can use the grated zest of half a lemon.

Pack your jar with the red onions and peel or zest.

To make the brine, put the sugar, apple cider vinegar, and salt into a small saucepan over a low heat until it reaches a gentle simmer. Immediately remove from the heat and let the sugar dissolve.

When the brine has cooled slightly (it doesn't need to be room temperature), pour it over the onions, ensuring that the brine completely covers them. If there's any extra brine that doesn't fit into your jar, keep it for a new pickle.

Keep the jar at room temperature; the onions will be ready to eat within an hour. I think they are best after 24 hours after which they should be moved to the fridge. They will keep indefinitely.

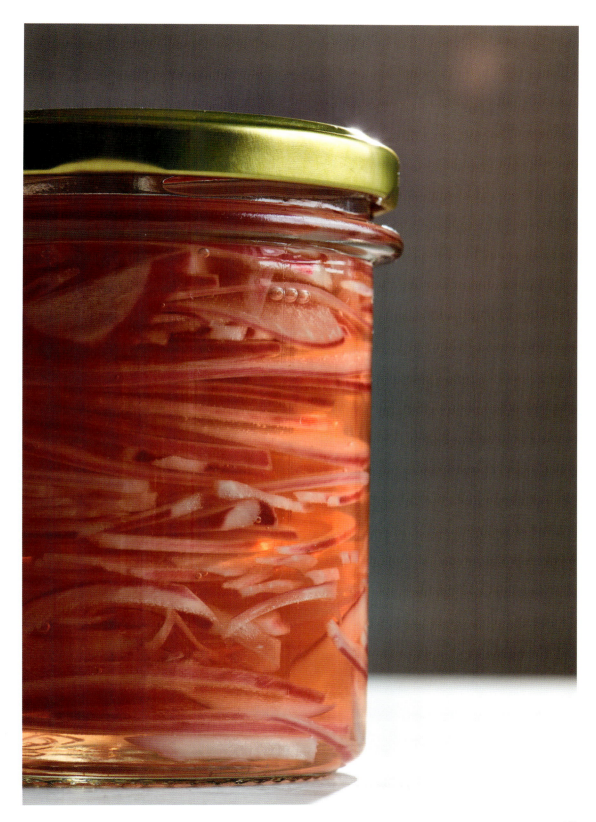

CRUNCHY SOY SAUCE CUCUMBERS

This is one of my favorite everyday Japanese pickles, with a combination of soy sauce and vinegar as its mode of preservation. Variations on this pickle were a constant in my childhood: eaten alongside rice balls and fried chicken during family road trips and always making an appearance at temple potlucks. They're the definition of delicious and all you really need to appreciate them is some rice to act as a canvas.

One important note here regards the types of cucumbers to use. I tend to go for baby cucumbers (about 6–10cm/2½–4in long) as these have less water content than the larger English variety. If you can get your hands on pickling cucumbers, those are ideal. Another non-negotiable here is using a Japanese soy sauce—other versions may have a different salt content and flavor. Like it spicy? Add more chiles. Also, the sugar content can be reduced if you want, but remember that the Japanese palate leans sweet. *See photo on the next page.*

PREP TIME: 20 MINUTES + minimum 2 hours salting

Makes one 1-liter (1-quart) jar

- 600g (1lb 5oz) small cucumbers
- 1 tsp salt
- 3 tbsp soy sauce
- 3 tbsp mirin
- 3 tbsp sugar
- 3 tbsp apple cider vinegar or, more traditionally, rice vinegar
- 1 whole dried chile, thinly sliced or cut with scissors
- 10g (0.33oz) fresh ginger, peeled and julienned

Cut each cucumber into fifths, about 1cm (½in) in size. Put these into a large bowl, add the salt, and mix thoroughly. Leave for a minimum of 2 hours or overnight. Try to stir regularly to ensure it's salted uniformly. The salting process will draw out liquid and allow the flavored brine to better infuse the vegetables.

After the salting period, discard the liquid from the cucumbers.

To make the brine, put all the remaining ingredients in a small saucepan and bring to a simmer until the sugar has dissolved. While the brine is still warm, pour it over the cucumbers. Transfer them to a glass jar for fridge storage.

You can eat them immediately but they are best after a day or two in the brine. The cucumbers will continue to emit water, so aim to eat them within 2 weeks.

KOMBUCHA-PICKLED CARROT & DAIKON

You're probably familiar with this sweet, crunchy, and colorful pickle often seen in Vietnamese cuisine, but did you know you can swap the vinegar for particularly sour over-fermented kombucha?

Any kombucha maker will commiserate over the woes of over-fermented kombucha, which can easily happen if you start to neglect it. For many people, this is the moment they give up on this fermented drink as they don't want overly sour kombucha. Fair enough, but why not use it as the acidic component for this pickle? The right level of acidity is vital for long-term preservation when making vinegar-based pickles, but as this one is kept in the fridge, kombucha works perfectly, especially if it's otherwise destined for the drain. While any flavor of kombucha will technically work here, I'd suggest going for plain (after the first fermentation), or a kombucha flavored with complementary aromatics, such as Ginger, Honey & Lemon (see page 131).

Any proportion of carrot to daikon will work and, as I like a bit of spice, I've added some mild green chile—you can use other chiles, fresh or dried. The brine is quite simple: It follows the 3:2:1 proportions of three parts acid (here, kombucha), two parts water, and one part sugar. *See photo on the next page.*

PREP TIME: 30 MINUTES | PICKLING TIME: 24 HOURS

Makes one 1-liter (1-quart) jar

375ml (1½ cups plus 1 tbsp) kombucha (alternatively use vinegar)
100g (3.5oz) sugar
1 tbsp salt
1 mild green chile, thinly sliced—more if you want it spicy!
400g (14oz) carrot, peeled
500g (1lb 2oz) daikon radish (mooli), peeled

In a small saucepan, gently warm the kombucha together with 240ml (1 cup) water, the sugar, salt, and green chile. Once the sugar has dissolved, remove the pan from the heat and leave the brine to infuse with the chile until it is lukewarm.

While the brine cools, julienne the carrot and daikon radish. A mandoline with a julienne blade is useful here, but if you're doing this by hand, ensure that the matchsticks are uniform in size, so that the vegetables pickle at the same rate.

Put the daikon and carrots into a jar and fill it with the brine. Leave overnight at room temperature and then transfer to the fridge. They will be ready to eat after 24 hours and are best consumed within 1 month.

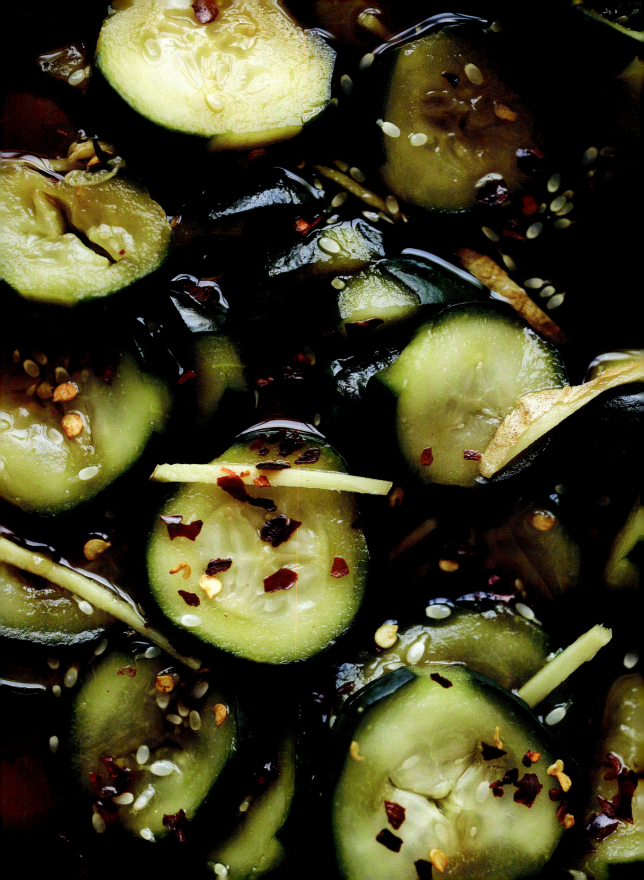

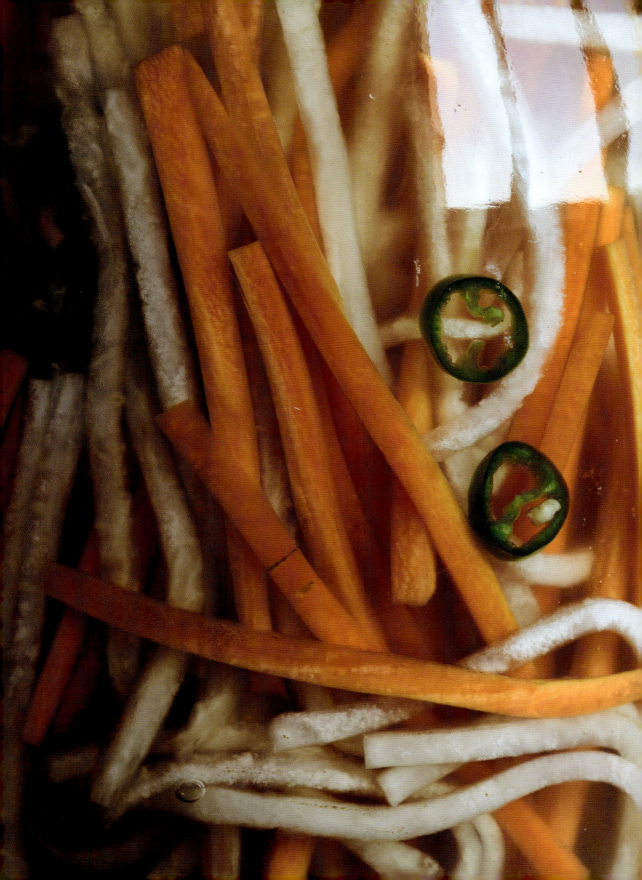

PICKLED FRUIT, THREE WAYS

Pickled fruit may sound odd, but think about all of the savory-leaning fruit chutneys and preserves. In many ways, pickled fruit actually seems quite obvious and is such a great way to preserve various fruits at the peak of their seasons. As with all pickling practices, you can get creative with the fruit and aromatics you use; my suggestion would be to stick with slightly harder fruit, as it'll be more resilient with the warm brine.

Pickled fruits are great with cheese (for example in my Pickled Fruit Tart with Goat Cheese, see page 163), and are also excellent alongside grilled meats, on salads, or in dressings (see Bitter Greens Salad with Pickled Pear Vinaigrette on page 186), and even in sweet recipes. *See photos on the next page.*

The three recipes below all follow the same process and proportions for their brine, and will each make one 500-ml (1-pint) jar. They take around 30 minutes to make. They are best enjoyed after 3 days and will keep indefinitely in the fridge.

PICKLED PLUMS WITH STAR ANISE & PINK PEPPERCORNS

- 3 plums (about 250g/9oz), pitted and cut into eighths
- 50g (1.75oz) sugar
- 180ml (¾ cup) apple cider vinegar
- 1½ tsp salt
- 2 star anise
- ½ tsp pink peppercorns

Prepare the fruit and put it in a jar.

To make the brine, put the sugar, apple cider vinegar, 120ml (½ cup) water, and salt into a small saucepan. Add the aromatics. Put the pan over a low heat until the liquid reaches a gentle simmer. Immediately remove from the heat and let the sugar dissolve and aromatics infuse the brine.

When the brine has cooled slightly (it doesn't need to be room temperature), pour it over the fruit, ensuring that the brine completely covers the pieces.

If there's any extra brine that doesn't fit into your jar, keep it for a new pickle.

Keep the jar at room temperature for 24 hours and then transfer it to the fridge for long-term storage.

PICKLED PEARS WITH THYME, CHILE & CORIANDER

1½ pears (about 250g/9oz), cored and cut into sixths
50g (1.75oz) sugar
180ml (¾ cup) apple cider vinegar
1½ tsp salt
2 sprigs of fresh thyme
1 mild chile, finely sliced, deseeded
½ tsp coriander seeds

Follow the method on page 120.

PICKLED GRAPES WITH GINGER & ALLSPICE

250g (9oz) grapes
50g (1.75oz) sugar
180ml (¾ cup) apple cider vinegar
1½ tsp salt
7g (0.25oz) fresh ginger, peeled and julienned
6 allspice berries

Follow the method on page 120.

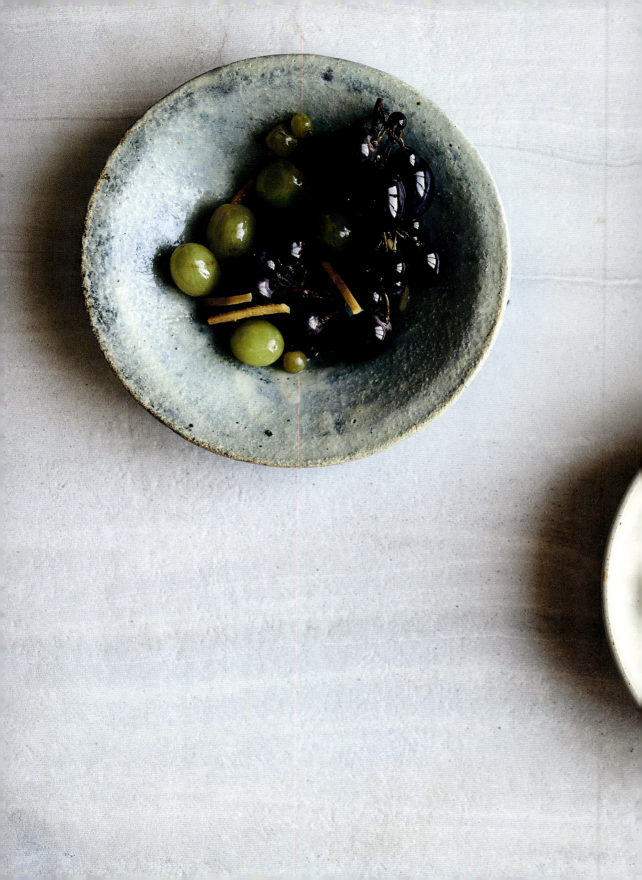

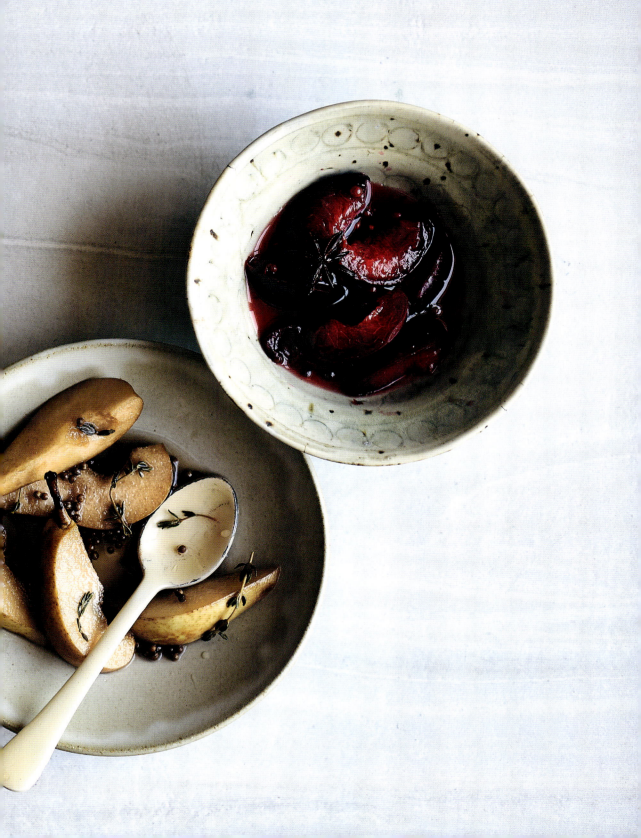

KOMBUCHA

There are a myriad of fermented drinks to explore in your home kitchen, from ginger bugs and natural sodas (where wild yeasts act as the starter for a fizzy drink) to water kefir, kvass, and kanji—three fermented drinks I make regularly whose origins span the globe from Eastern Europe to South Asia. One of the challenges in writing this book was the need to focus: Metaphorical lines in the sand must be drawn, otherwise there are just too many rabbit holes to explore. While this is a good problem to have, let's pivot to another "K" on this alliterative list and perhaps the one most familiar to you: kombucha, the fermented tea.

My relationship with kombucha started back in college and came out of a desire not for health, nor an interest in fermentation (shocker!), but as a way to use up my seemingly endless campus dining points, a problem for many of us with an on-campus dining plan. It was the early 2010s and the American kombucha market appeared to be monopolized by one player, pioneering a fermented tea drink to the masses and branding it through an aspirational lens: tasteful typography, distinct and sturdy glass bottles, and the then novel use of now common buzzwords. This brand of kombucha was expensive, so by buying bottles, I quickly maxed out my monthly dining points. This isn't to say that I didn't love the sour tang and slightly effervescent drink, but it also ticked many of the boxes I sought when buying drinks to fill my dorm mini-fridge. I have a penchant for low-sugar drinks and an enduring love for cold tea, and it was ultimately new and different.

I lived my life in organized chaos (and continue to do so, as my husband will attest to). Clean, yes, but messy, and my dorm room reflected this. Textbooks and notebooks strewn among a rainbow of Post-it notes, and emerging from this landscape, bottles of kombucha destined for the recycling bin: an inch or two remaining, lids slightly ajar, and upon closer inspection, the start of something magical—although I did not know that then.

What was this gunky creature in my kombucha? Stringy, jellyfish-like, and growing quickly in the warmth of my dorm room, I assumed it was a sure sign that the kombucha was off. And when I dared try tasting it? Phlegm-like slime. Excuse my immaturity as a late teen, but this reaction isn't uncommon to those new to this ferment. But to those familiar with this wonderful fermented drink, you'll know I was witnessing the early formation of the pellicle, also known as the kombucha SCOBY (Symbiotic Culture Of Bacteria and Yeast), in the fermented kombucha, aka the kombucha starter.

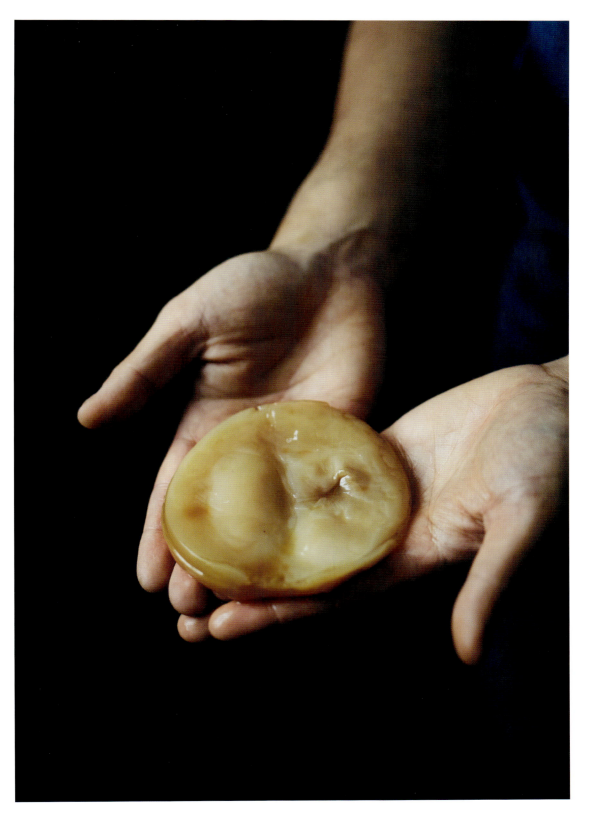

While technically all you need to make kombucha is the starter tea (as I learned in my dorm room), the pellicle helps greatly, with both components driving the fermentation: consuming the sugar in the tea and creating an acidic, tangy, and slightly effervescent drink. I often compare this to making sourdough at home; you can make a sourdough starter from scratch or use a starter to accelerate and guarantee its success. Instead of flour and water, you're using tea and sugar to feed the SCOBY to create kombucha. This is what is generally called the first fermentation; your kombucha is completed, albeit unflavored, and you should have a new pellicle floating at the top of your kombucha.

SCOBY pellicles can come in all shapes and sizes, from floaty gel-like bits indicating positive signs of live cultures, to large gelatinous disks, akin to vinegar mothers but made of different bacteria and yeast. Kombucha is the fermented gift that keeps on giving, with each successful batch producing a new pellicle. Anyone who makes kombucha will have run into the problem of having way too many SCOBY pellicles. Gift them to friends (alongside the starter liquid) to encourage them to join the kombucha party or keep them in a separate jar (often called a SCOBY hotel—see page 136), or compost them.

But what about the flavors, and how do you optimize fizzy effervescence? Well, that's what we call the secondary fermentation of kombucha and I'll dive into this in the recipes in this section, followed by my answers to some of the most common questions I encounter when making kombucha.

KOMBUCHA 101

There are two main steps when making kombucha: the first fermentation and second fermentation.

PREP TIME: 1 HOUR | FERMENTATION TIME: 12–19 DAYS

Makes 1 liter (1 quart) kombucha

- 2 black tea bags (or 1½ tsp loose leaf tea)
- 50g (1.75oz) granulated sugar
- 120–240ml (½–1 cup) kombucha starter liquid and gel-like pellicle

SPECIAL EQUIPMENT: 1.5-liter (1.5-quart) glass jar; 1-liter (1-quart) glass swing-top bottle; breathable cotton cloth

FIRST FERMENTATION

Put the tea and sugar in a large pan. Boil 1 liter (1 quart) of water and pour it over the tea and sugar. Let the sugar dissolve and the tea infuse for 30–45 minutes. Do not do this step directly in your glass jar in case it can't handle the heat.

If you want to scale up the kombucha to make larger batches, make a concentrated sweet tea and dilute it with cold water to speed up the process, but ensure that you have sufficient starter liquid for a successful batch while maintaining the correct proportions.

Remove the tea bags (or strain the sweetened tea into a clean container if using loose leaf) and leave until cool to the touch (not lukewarm). If the liquid is too warm it can kill the necessary bacteria.

Add the starter liquid and the pellicle to the jar. The pellicle will have a mind of its own and may float or sink—don't worry too much about this.

Cover the jar with a breathable cotton cloth and secure it with a rubber band. Let this ferment out of direct sunlight and in an environment with relatively stable temperatures between 60–80°F (16–27°C). I make kombucha throughout the year and at varying temperatures: This just means that fermentation may take more or less time.

The first fermentation may take between 7–14 days, during which you may witness the color of the tea changing slightly as well as some yeast and bacterial growth giving the kombucha its characteristic cloudy appearance. Remember that a new pellicle or additional yeast and bacterial growth is a sign of success. More importantly, taste the kombucha after that initial week. If it still tastes like sweet tea (and nothing else), let it continue fermenting. If it's slightly sour, effervescent, and tasting like kombucha, your first ferment is done! As your confidence and awareness of these signs grow, this first step will become intuitive.

The kombucha is now completed and you can do one of two things: enjoy it as is (I love unflavored kombucha) or start the second fermentation.

SECOND FERMENTATION

A lot of the fun with kombucha is in its second fermentation. Bottling the kombucha after the first fermentation is what gives kombucha its effervescence. This is because a closed system allows for carbon dioxide to build up as the microbes continue to consume sugar. The advantages of flavoring the kombucha include not only making it more palatable for those new to this fermented drink, but also adding an additional source of sugar which will result in increased carbonation.

At this point, many recipes will suggest adding the flavoring ingredients directly to the bottle. However, I find this can get a bit messy, so I first infuse the ingredients with the kombucha (once the starter liquid and pellicle have been removed) before bottling it up.

Remove the gel-like pellicle and 120–240ml (½–1 cup) of the kombucha and reserve as the starter liquid for your next batch.

In the same jar, add your flavors of choice (see pages 130–131 for some of my favorites). Leave to infuse for 2 days at room temperature, covered with a breathable cotton cloth.

After 2 days, strain out the added ingredients (which generally lack flavor; I usually compost everything). After this infusion, you may even notice the initial growth of a new pellicle, which can be added to the final bottle.

Decant the infused kombucha into a 1-liter (1-quart) swing-top bottle, leaving around 2.5cm (1in) headspace at the top. Secure the bottle's lid and leave to ferment at room temperature for 2–3 days. Once bottled up, the kombucha enters its second fermentation. During this period, you should notice bubbling as well as more pellicle and yeast growth, similar to the first fermentation. After this point, transfer it to the fridge and enjoy!

As the microbes continue to consume sugars and create carbon dioxide within a closed bottle, it can be an active ferment. The timing and the ingredients you add in the second ferment directly impact the levels of carbonation. I urge you to be careful to avoid the risk of exploding bottles. This has never happened to me, but it's not unusual for bottles to overflow with carbonation when opening them. If you are nervous about this, keep the bottles in the fridge before opening (or open them outside). I therefore wouldn't recommend fermenting kombucha in a closed bottle at room temperature for more than 2–3 days. You can burp your bottles to release pressure, but this will also reduce the carbonation you may want in the final drink. I suggest making small batches and keeping them in the fridge, which eases the pressure build-up.

Kombucha is about personal taste. As you make and drink more often, take note of your preferences and adjust the process accordingly.

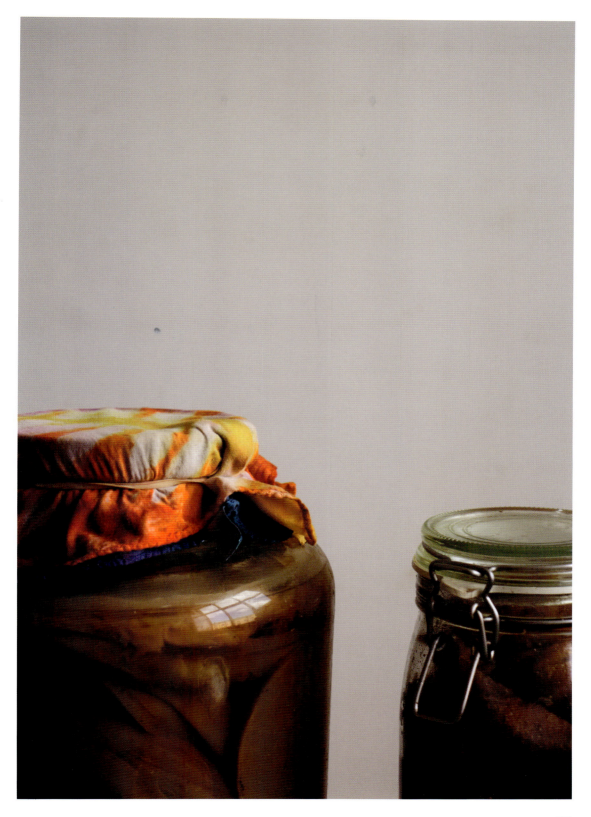

KOMBUCHA, FIVE WAYS

FERMENTS

FROZEN BERRIES & HIBISCUS

100g (3.5oz) frozen mixed berries (or any combination of frozen raspberries, strawberries, blueberries, etc.)
pinch of dried hibiscus leaves

This kombucha is dark, sweet, and slightly earthy due to the hibiscus. I like to use frozen fruit for the second fermentation as the kombucha extracts the flavor well as it defrosts. This is also a nice lesson in showing how an ingredient that is processed (frozen berries, dried hibiscus) can impart flavor. *See photos on the next page.*

MANGO & CHILI

150g (5oz) frozen mango
¼ tsp chili powder

This is the first kombucha I make when warm weather hits. I don't like to "waste" fresh mangoes during their short season for flavoring kombucha; frozen mango is a much easier (and cheaper) option. Frozen fruit is generally frozen at its peak ripeness so it should be sweet but is nicely balanced with dried chili powder. *See photos on the next page.*

GINGER, HONEY & LEMON

50g (1.75oz) fresh ginger, skin left on, thinly sliced

1 lemon, thinly sliced

1 tbsp honey

This is a classic flavor combination and for a good reason. Who doesn't love the comfort of tea, ginger, honey, and lemon? As you'd expect, this translates to a slightly fiery kombucha thanks to the ginger. Best yet, you probably have all of the ingredients needed for this in your pantry. *See photos on the next page.*

BLUEBERRY & ROSEMARY

150g (5oz) blueberries, gently mashed

2 sprigs of fresh rosemary, roughly chopped or bashed

The flavor of herbs comes through beautifully in kombucha: Varieties of mint and basil work well, but rosemary is particularly herbaceous and woody, resulting in a really interesting and complex drink. *See photos on the next page.*

CHEONG

150ml (½ cup plus 2 tbsp) cheong (any variety, see page 142)

All varieties of cheong work nicely for the second kombucha fermentation, as they include a lot of sugar and the extracted fruit flavor. I tend to use a combination of both the cheong syrup and the preserved fruit, but if you can't be bothered to strain the fruit out at the end, just use the syrup.

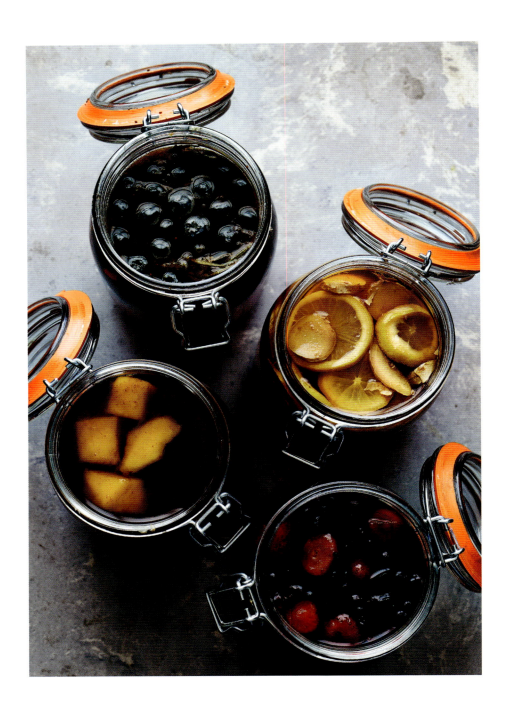

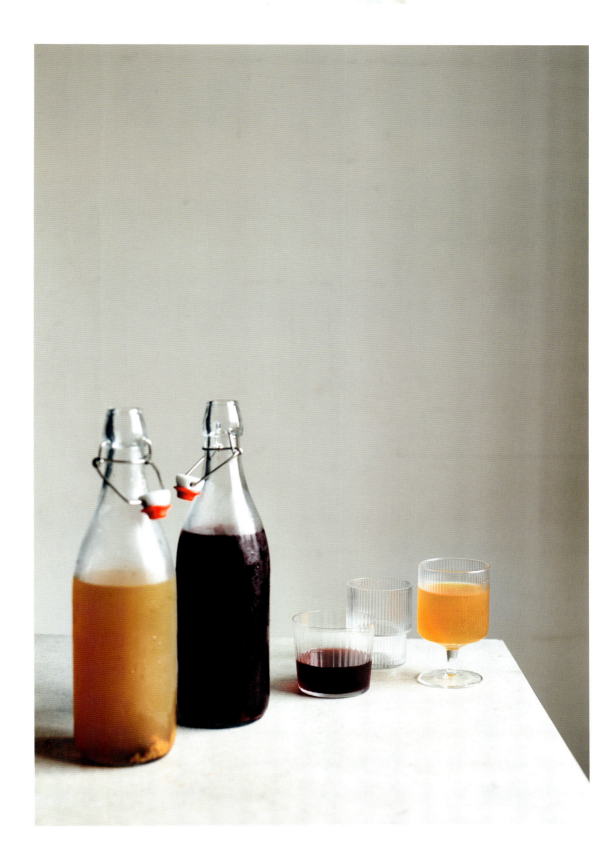

Q&A

As outlined in the Kombucha 101 method (see page 127), there are many variables at play when making kombucha to your individual liking. I have found that there are lots of questions people have for this very reason—which is true for the entire life cycle of kombucha. Below are some of the most common questions I encounter.

Where do I find a SCOBY or pellicle?

Remember that you really just need the starter liquid (fermented kombucha), as I learned when I was in college. But a pellicle is great to have and, in my opinion, does increase the likelihood of success. Ask friends and neighborhood groups—I guarantee you'll find someone who makes kombucha and is eager to get rid of a pellicle and some of their starter liquid. You can also buy both the starter liquid and pellicle online, which may be faster than coordinating with friends. Or make your own, as follows:

400ml (1⅔ cup) unpasteurized kombucha, ideally unflavored

In a glass jar, cover the kombucha with a breathable lid and secure it with a rubber band.

Leave to ferment out of direct sunlight and at room temperature for 3–6 weeks. The time needed will depend on the temperature at which you're fermenting, so the exact time could be shorter or longer.

Check the kombucha every week. The kombucha will start to evaporate and there should be some pellicle growth, potentially looking like a gel-like disc or, if it's younger, jellyfish-like strands of growth. Once the pellicle is around 5mm (¼in) in thickness, living in rather acidic kombucha, you're ready to start your first batch with this new pellicle and the starter liquid.

Can I use different types of tea or sugar?

I'd always suggest starting your kombucha journey with black tea. However, as your confidence grows and your starter liquid and pellicles mature, you can definitely change it up with combinations of tea—I often like a 50:50 blend of black and green tea.

Sugar alternatives will not work—the bacteria and yeast consume sugar for the kombucha's fermentation. Honey can be used, but for a different fermented drink known as "jun"; however, this requires a few batches to train the starter liquid and pellicle to consume honey.

What type of breathable lid should I use for the first fermentation?

Any breathable cotton cloth or kitchen towel will work well. As this is an aerobic process—meaning that it requires oxygen—the kombucha needs to be exposed to the air. The breathable lid keeps out any debris and fruit flies. Some resources suggest using muslin or cheesecloth, but I find this to not be ideal as pesky fruit flies can easily get through those holes.

What about contact with metal? Isn't that bad for fermentation and kombucha?

Most recipes for kombucha will tell you that any contact with metal is a no-go as it can be detrimental to the starter liquid and the end product. This is usually only a real concern if the kombucha has long exposure to the metal. In the home kitchen setting, using the occasional metal spoon or funnel will not hurt your kombucha.

Nothing is happening! What went wrong?

If you follow process on pages 127–28, the usual culprit is temperature: If the environment is too cold, the starter liquid can go dormant and will inhibit how acidic the kombucha gets, which could lead to unwanted mold growth. Conversely, if it's too hot (either the initial tea or the environment's temperature), this will also inhibit microbial growth, leading to mold.

I'm not getting carbonation during my second fermentation. How do I increase this?

While it's possible to see some effervescence during a kombucha's first fermentation, carbonation is usually created in a closed bottle during its second fermentation as the microbes continue to consume sugar and produce carbon dioxide. As this is a natural process, there are several things you can try to increase carbonation:

—Add fresh ingredients and more sugar to accelerate microbial activity.

—Ensure your bottles are airtight—swing-top bottles are my go-to bottles for the second fermentation, as they're built for this pressure.

—Don't open/burp your bottles, and after the initial fermentation at room temperature, move them to the fridge. Burping your bottles allows all gas build-up to dissipate.

What is continuous kombucha brewing?

Unlike making a batch of kombucha, as in the process outlined earlier, continuous brewing is a non-stop method for the first fermentation, and the main method of brewing kombucha I do at home. This is really suggested only if you make large batches of kombucha, continuously, allowing you to have a steady source of kombucha completed up to its first fermentation. You then simply decant the completed kombucha from the continuous brew, ready for the flavor infusion and second fermentation. Replace the decanted kombucha with equal parts of sweetened tea, as the remaining kombucha acts as the starter liquid. There is a risk that the kombucha from a continuous brew can over-ferment and become too sour; however, this can still be used as a starter liquid for fresh batches. Just be sure that you're constantly feeding the continuous brew with new sweetened tea so it doesn't get too sour and also does not evaporate.

What is a SCOBY hotel?

A SCOBY hotel is the slightly silly (but descriptive) name given to your store of pellicles and starter liquid. If you're continuously brewing kombucha, the container holding your continuous brew can act as the SCOBY hotel, but the purpose of a SCOBY hotel is to hold extra pellicles in a safe environment when you're not actively making kombucha. I tend to put all bacterial and yeast growth—from the gel-like layers to the stringy bits of yeast—in my SCOBY hotel when not using them. You need to feed the hotel regularly with sweetened tea as the kombucha can evaporate and you do not want the pellicles to dry out. I like to keep my hotels sealed with an airtight lid to minimize evaporation. Pellicles are highly durable, so feel free to cut them so they fit your hotel; however, be sure you're using pellicles only from the first fermentation, before flavorings are added. If you do decide to use your pellicles with other flavorings, keep these separate so they don't potentially contaminate the SCOBY hotel. Don't neglect your SCOBY hotel: Aim to check in monthly and top up if needed with either sweetened tea or fermented kombucha (after the first fermentation). And if you have too many pellicles? Compost them, or give them to friends to continue the kombucha life cycle.

My kombucha is too sour! What do I do with over-fermented kombucha?

This is a common woe but is not a bad thing—if it happens after the first fermentation, you should still be able to create a delicious batch of kombucha after adding the additional flavors, although it could obviously lean sour. For some, this may be exactly what you want, but if you lean sweeter, add additional sources of sugar in the second fermentation. Regardless if it's the first or second fermentation, however, a sour kombucha can be used in so many different ways: Dilute it with soda water and drink it over ice, use it in dressings instead of vinegar or lemon, or even use it as a starter liquid for other fun kitchen projects, such as the Kombucha Citrus Syrup (see page 138).

KOMBUCHA CITRUS SYRUP

This recipe and its origin exemplify what I've loved most about my journey through fermentation: the cross-cultural and global connections, both with food and friends. One of my first friends on social media was Payal Shah. She taught me an endless amount, but her ethos surrounding fermentation and its treatment in a home setting ignited such a passion in me. And I just love that a friend living in India stretched my mind by using kombucha to help ferment a Korean cheong; and here I am in London writing about it, one of the most important ingredients in my fermentation larder.

In principle, this is a riff on a cheong, a fermented fruit syrup from Korea, but it uses kombucha as a starter liquid to accelerate the fermentation. Due to the amount of sugar it's hard to get this process wrong, but the beauty of this recipe truly shines as this syrup continuously evolves. For more information on cheong, please see page 142.

Throw in your skinless lemons from martini making, or your unused lime wedges from last night's dinner. Just remember to top it up with sugar (most important) and occasionally with kombucha, which will always kickstart some microbial activity. Stick to the proportions in the recipe opposite as a guideline for topping up this ferment as it matures. My batch has been continuously fermenting at room temperature in a beautifully preserved state since 2020, so if you stick to the best practices in this book, yours too can last a long time. *See photos on the next page.*

PREP TIME: 10 MINUTES
WAIT TIME: minimum 2–3 WEEKS

Makes one 500-ml (1-pint) jar

approximately 300g (10.5oz) citrus fruit (for example 1 orange, 1 lemon, and 1 lime), thinly sliced

approximately 300g (10.5oz) sugar (use the same amount as the weight of your citrus fruit)

1 tbsp unpasteurized kombucha

Place the citrus fruit in a bowl and add an equal amount of sugar. Mix together to encourage the sugar to dissolve. Mix in your kombucha and transfer it all to a jar, packing it down to minimize oxygen and air pockets.

During the first week, give the jar an occasional shake, until all of the sugar has dissolved. The sugar will draw out the liquid from the citrus so you should soon have a syrup. You can technically start using this ingredient immediately, but I recommend tasting it every month, observing the changing flavors. The syrup will keep indefinitely in the fridge.

How can I use kombucha citrus syrup?

—Use it as a sweetener for dressings or marinades wherever honey or sugar is required; this works particularly well with Mediterranean and East Asian flavor profiles and, when mixed with soy sauce, makes a delicious ponzu dressing.

—It acts well as a glaze for sweet custard or fruit pies, or for roasts (such as a Christmas ham).

—Mix it with drinks—from summer cocktails to mulled wine—whenever citrus and sugar is needed.

—Use it as the flavoring and source of sugar in kombucha during its second fermentation.

—Use the preserved fruit in desserts, blitzed into a marmalade-like jam for topping yogurt.

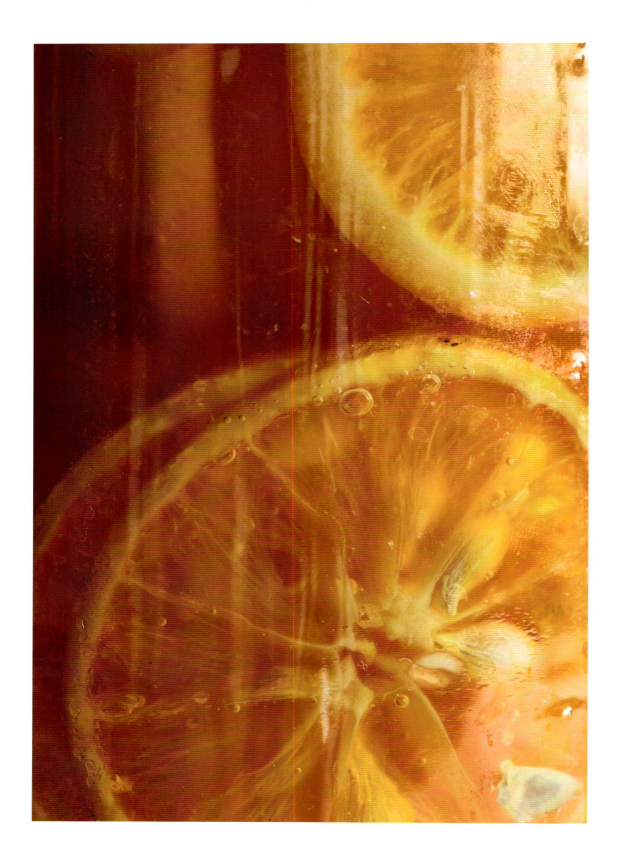

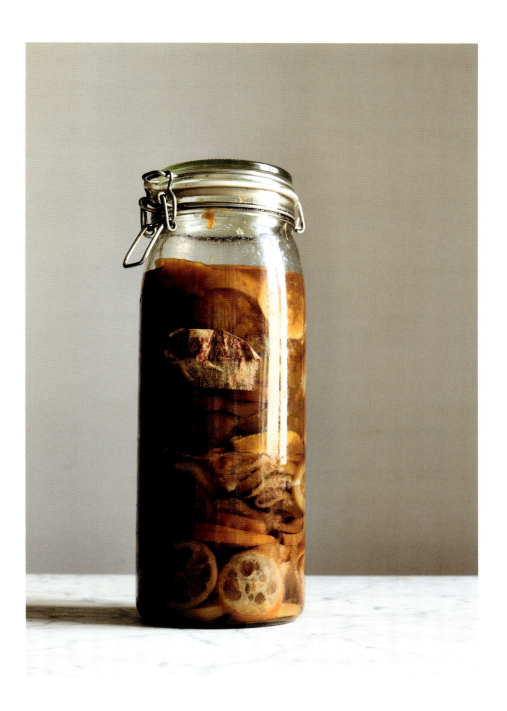

CHEONG

Cheong is one of my latest preoccupations, particularly as an answer to reduce waste in the kitchen and a way to capture seasonal flavors. It is a Korean preservation technique where equal parts sugar and fruit are mixed together and preserved as the sugar extracts liquid from the fruit: You're left with a sweet syrup, intensely flavored by the fruit you're using, and the equally delicious preserved fruit.

In Korea, whole green plums are generally used and once the cheong is complete, the shrivelled fruit is strained out and used to make plum wine or mixed with savory ingredients in side dishes. In Korean cuisine, maesil (plum) cheong is often used as a sweetener in savory dishes—which I'd recommend. However, I tend to use cheong primarily in sweet dishes. And if you need a simple syrup for a cocktail? Replace it with a cheong.

My approach is slightly different but honors the traditional technique. Cutting the fruit into small pieces increases the surface area and allows for the sugar to extract water more quickly. You'll want to minimize the fruit's exposure to oxygen as this can attract unwanted yeast; a fermentation weight (or a piece of plastic wrap or parchment paper sitting on top of the cheong to act as a barrier between the liquid/fruit and oxygen) will minimize the risk.

Here is my general process, followed by a few of my favorite cheong flavors; the "recipe" remains the same, no matter how much produce you're using. As with most of my methodology in this book, you can get creative—mix up fruit or vegetable combinations and throw in spices (apples and cinnamon, anyone?)—as long as you stick to the basic process. In my experience most sugar varieties will work, however, the type can impact the final flavor profile (i.e., brown or demerara will go darker and lead to a deeper flavor); I would not recommend using sugar alternatives as this could impact the liquid extraction process and therefore the final cheong product.

Treat the final product as two separate ingredients: a delicious syrup for both sweet and savory recipes, and preserved fruit—sometimes preserved with textural structure, as with rhubarb and cucumbers, and sometimes as a compote, with a jammy consistency, as with the plums and mixed berries. When it comes to cheong making, the only limit is your imagination.

CHEONG 101

PREP TIME: 15 MINUTES (or more, depending on quantity)
WAIT TIME: 2-3 WEEKS, but can continue indefinitely

fruit, or vegetables with high water content, chopped into small pieces
sugar

Place the prepared fruit or vegetables in a bowl, and using a kitchen scale, weigh the amount and add an equal amount of sugar. Mix together to encourage the sugar to dissolve. Use a spatula to decant everything into a glass jar, ensuring you scrape in all the residual sugar.

Leave the jar at room temperature. Over the next few days, the sugar should begin extracting water from the produce. It is likely that sugar will gather at the bottom of the jar. If so, turn it upside down or shake it vigorously to encourage the sugar to dissolve. You could use a clean spoon to mix the liquid but I don't to avoid potential contamination.

Once most of the sugar has dissolved (usually within 5 days) and the fruit or vegetables are floating in liquid, you can add a fermentation weight or a piece of parchment paper on top of the liquid to minimize its contact with oxygen. It's not uncommon for there to be slight oxidation of the fruit or vegetables (you may see a change in color), but as long as there's no mold or white blooms of yeast, it should be fine. Yeast will be attracted to fruit protruding from the liquid, so make sure everything is submerged (as "everything is fine below the brine").

You can start using the cheong after around 2-3 weeks and at this point you have a few options:

—Use the syrup in desserts, dressings, and drinks. Strain out the fruit and serve with yogurt, add to baked goods, or infuse with alcohol.

—Move the cheong (either strained or with fruit left in) to the fridge: This will slow down any microbial activity.

—Leave the fruit in and let the flavors continue to evolve at room temperature: This is usually what I do, as I find the flavors really change throughout a cheong's life cycle. The cheong may get a bit effervescent, or even slightly alcohol-like in taste, which can lead to even more interesting usages in the kitchen.

It can last indefinitely, especially in the fridge. I have batches of cheong (both strained and with the fruit in it) that are nearly a year old.

CHEONG, FOUR WAYS

FERMENTS

RHUBARB

fresh rhubarb, cut into thin (about 5-mm/ ¼-inch) slices
sugar

Rhubarb was a new flavor for me in my adulthood, but it became a favorite after I moved to London. In this new home I became much more aware of seasonality, and with that came a sense of excitement as the seasons changed and new produce emerged in farmers markets and on supermarket shelves. There are so many ways to capture the flavor of rhubarb—from jams and chutneys to pickles and ferments—but cheong is one of my favorites. It extracts such a lovely flavor from the rhubarb and also retains its crunch, giving us the best of both worlds. I've used this cheong in the Preserved Rhubarb & Mixed Berry Pound Cake (see page 242) and as a topping for a Rhubarb Cheong Pavlova (see page 245), but I guarantee you'll find endless uses for it at home.

MIXED BERRY

frozen mixed berries
sugar

While you can make cheong from fresh berries, frozen mixed berries are an excellent choice. As the fruit thaws, it accelerates the cheong-making process similarly to using frozen fruit to flavor a kombucha. The main thing to note here is that, as the fruit is already "processed" through being frozen and then defrosting, it could lead to a more lively cheong that potentially even starts to ferment within 2 weeks. This isn't a bad thing: It might taste slightly effervescent or even a little alcoholic, both of which get muted if you cook with this cheong. No preparation is needed: Just dump the frozen fruit into your glass jar with the sugar.

PLUM

fresh plums, pitted and cut into eighths
sugar
fresh thyme sprigs (optional)

This cheong was a happy accident born out of failure. One of my first preservation projects many years ago was making umeshu, or plum wine. I struggled to find the correct green, tart, almost inedible plums needed for the recipe, so I bought several pounds of dark purple plums to see what would happen. Luckily I had the foresight to make only a small batch, because it didn't work too well. So, with a large amount of plums needing a home, I turned to cheong and ended up creating what is now a staple in my preservation larder. This method works with all stone fruit varieties, including sour plums, peaches, apricots, and cherries. If using apricots, cut them into quarters, and if using cherries, halve them. You could leave the plums whole as in the traditional method for making Korean plum wine, but this will require significantly longer to make the syrup (3–4 months minimum).

CUCUMBER

fresh cucumber, sliced as thinly as possible
sugar
fresh dill (optional)

Although traditionally made with fruit, cheong can be made with vegetables that have a high water content. A cucumber cheong immediately transports me to a perfect London summer day: a picnic on an open green with Pimm's in hand, a salad with just-picked produce from my urban garden, herbaceous and fresh. As you may have guessed, cucumber cheong is not only great in mixed drinks, it's also a source of sugar in summer salad dressing. And the leftover cucumber slices? Exciting garnishes with a hit of vegetable sweetness.

This method works with all varieties of cucumbers, as well as other high-water content vegetables, such as tomatoes, cut into equal-size small pieces to optimize surface area.

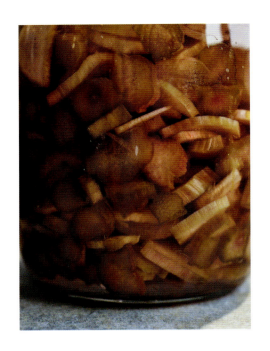
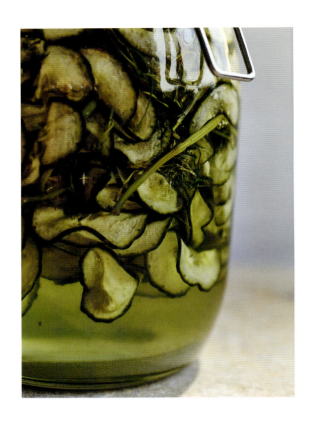
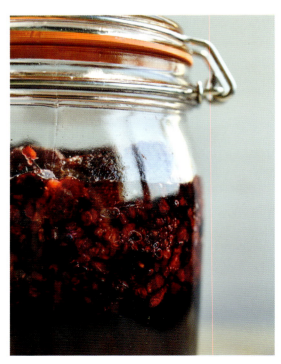

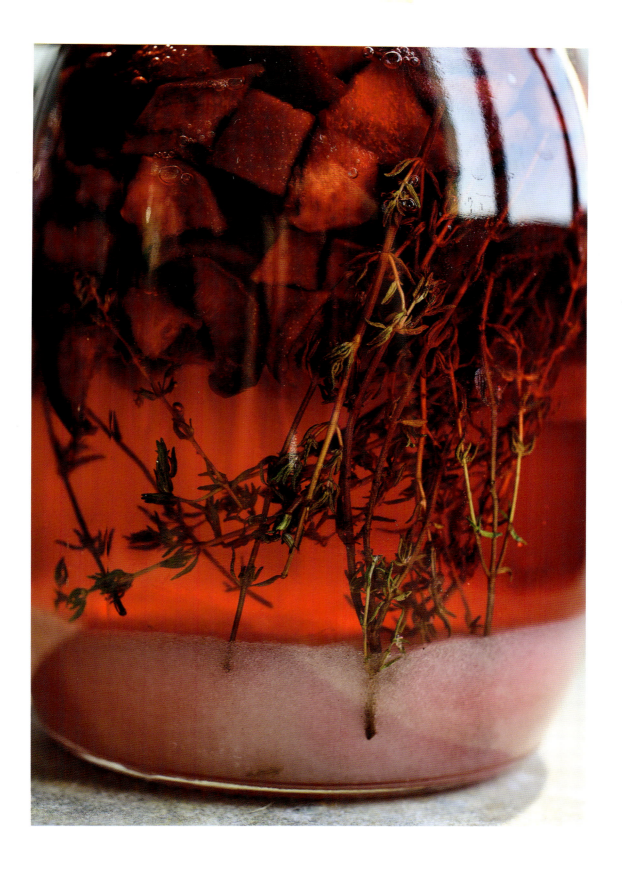

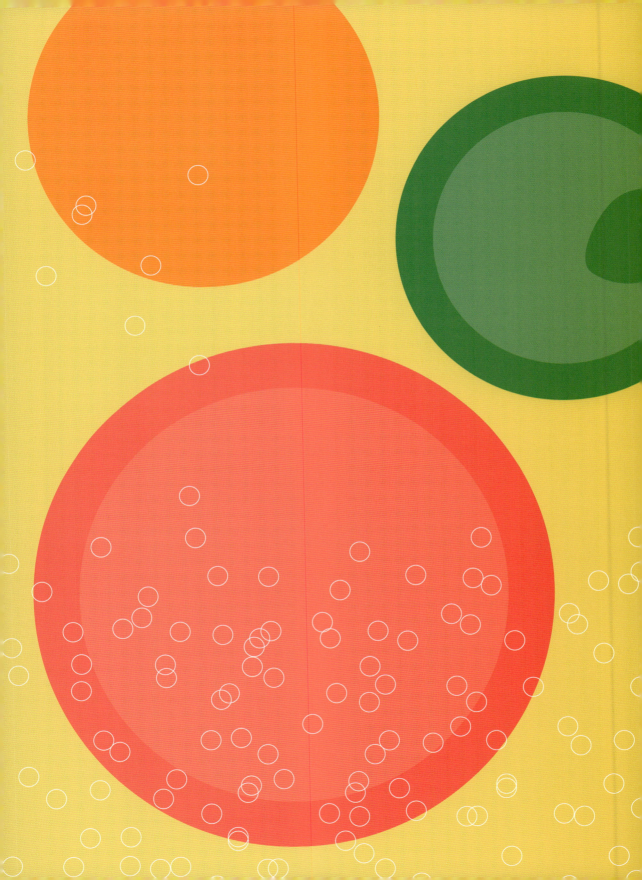

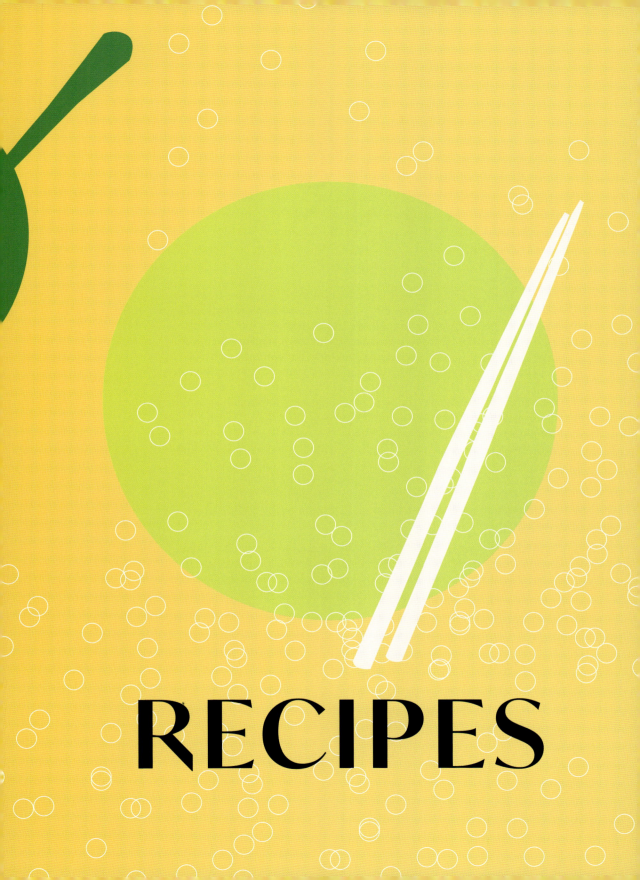

HOW TO COOK WITH PICKLES & FERMENTS

RECIPES

I like to think of using ferments and pickles in cooking like ripples in water, with each circle expanding outward as we explore potential flavors and uses. And it's in this exploration that you can balance elements: freshly fermented versus overly funky, layering tastes and textures, color and variety. Yes, a pickle or ferment can be appreciated in its own right, but I encourage you not to let these jars languish in your fridge or at the back of your pantry. The power of ferments and pickles lies in how they can be combined, showcasing not only their tremendous diversity but also how their flavors evolve when they are used in cooking. The next level of flavor is unlocked with the application of heat. The healthy bacteria may die, but what you're left with are building blocks of flavor which will turn even the simplest of meals into something special. You'll be hard-pressed to find a dish that can't happily incorporate some of the preserves explored in this book or be improved with the tangy crunch of a pickle.

In the following section, I'll share many of my favorite recipes that build on what I've learned through making and using preserves in different countries and creating my own food traditions in London.

A few notes on the recipes:

—I don't expect you to make every ferment or pickle in this book (although that would be very cool). You may be too busy or you may have a tried and tested version you'd prefer to use. I encourage you to use what you want. Commercially available alternatives will always work. In developing these recipes, I used homemade and therefore unpasteurized fermented products. Check the labels for terms such as "alive," "live cultures," or "raw," but generally speaking if they are in cold storage at the store, they are unpasteurized and more true to their origin. Pasteurized versions will include preservatives (such as vinegar), which add flavors, so the results might differ slightly.

—For recipes that use sauerkraut, I've aimed to keep the additional flavors at a minimum to allow for them to be somewhat interchangeable depending on the type of sauerkraut you're using.

—For recipes that use kimchi, I opt for older and more fermented cabbage-based kimchi: Its stronger flavor and softer texture lend itself better for cooking. Cabbage kimchi is also generally the most accessible commercially. When referring to "older" kimchi for cooking, any store-bought kimchi will work; if it's homemade, I would suggest waiting until it's fully fermented and the flavor and texture of the cabbage has changed. As a top tip, divide your homemade kimchi into two smaller batches, keeping one in the fridge to eat as kimchi, and leaving the second batch at room temperature to use in cooking.

—For recipes that use miso, I expect many of you will buy miso (versus making it from scratch)—the most readily accessible varieties being white and red miso. While these are different products, both are salty drivers of umami, so you could use them interchangeably; however, remember that white miso is less salty than red miso, so adjust other ingredients according to taste.

Does cooking destroy gut-loving bacteria?

One of the major pulls to fermenting in your home kitchen is its impact on your digestion, especially given today's focus on and increased awareness of gut health, probiotics, and prebiotics. Eating fermented and preserved Japanese pickles was a mainstay with meals, my grandparents reminding me to eat them alongside almost everything. I listened to their words of wisdom—not just because I wanted to be a good grandchild, but also because they tasted so darn great and it made me feel good after what was often a very filling meal. Diversity in what we eat—both fermented and otherwise—has a massive impact on our physical and mental well-being. Eat your favorite fermented products regularly for this reason, however, do not be afraid to cook them, with my recipes as your jumping-off point. Yes, the good bacteria will not survive the heat of many of the following recipes, but as I mentioned earlier, you're left with incredible flavor to explore.

STARTERS

Styling a Pickle Platter

A good pickle platter offers a diversity of color, texture, and flavor. As a child—and still to this day—my favorite element of a Japanese meal was the selection of pickles, as commonplace in bento boxes as it is in high-end multi-course meals. Besides acting as an aid to digestion, the selection of pickles generally would showcase different preservation techniques, textures, and colors, all of which are the ingredients that create an impactful pickle platter. It's also an excellent medium to show off your creativity and everything you're preserving at home (and who doesn't want the opportunity to show off?). This obviously requires some planning, but if you have this book, you're probably going to start amassing some jars of ferments and pickles. Or you may start buying more to learn what you like (and subsequently want to commit to learning)! A pickle platter is about impact, so go in with bold flavors ... which will hopefully result in a balanced approach to pickle varieties or a memorable dinner party! *See photo on the next page.*

- —Choose a **minimum of three pickles**. Two seems too few and will lead to immediate comparison. Be mindful not to overcrowd the plate with similar flavors in order for each pickle to be appreciated independently. Be mindful of what each pickle is offering and aim for a balance between salt, umami, sweetness, sourness, and heat.
- —**Variety is important**—not just in color but also preservation technique. Balance a sweet and sour **vinegar-based** bread and butter pickle beaming with yellow against funky **lactofermented** crudites in shades of green and the ombre reds of **kimchi**.

— Showcase different ages of a ferment, like vintages of a wine, through the **lens of texture**: Fresh kimchi has a crunch; older kimchi will be softer. Consider cutting them into smaller pieces to optimize the right hit of flavor.

— **Think beyond pickles**—why not include a spoonful of homemade miso or even miso varieties at different stages of fermentation? Preserved fruit from cheong or from making kombucha?

— Include **a shot of brine**. When you're consuming the pickles, don't forget about the brine. It's a fun addition to a pickle platter and great for a dinner party, especially if that brine is later used in cocktails (see pages 254–260).

Some of my go-to combinations are included below. I've used bold to highlight what's in the platter on the next page:

— Corner Store Kimchi (page 58), **Zucchini Bread & Butter Pickles** (page 109), **Gazpacho Cherry Tomatoes** (page 43)

— **Garam Masala Sauerkraut** (page 36), **Rhubarb Kimchi** (page 75), Crunchy Soy Sauce Cucumbers (page 116)

— Garlic Misozuke (page 97), Sour Dill Pickles (page 44), Chipotle & Carrot Sauerkraut (page 51)

You could enjoy pickle platters as they are, or serve them with foods that will act as a foil to the zingy flavors. Options include:

— Crackers or toasted sliced sourdough and soft creamy cheese

— Plain white rice or onigiri (rice balls)

— Thin slices of cucumber, whole radishes, celery— these are particularly good to serve alongside any miso or miso-like paste.

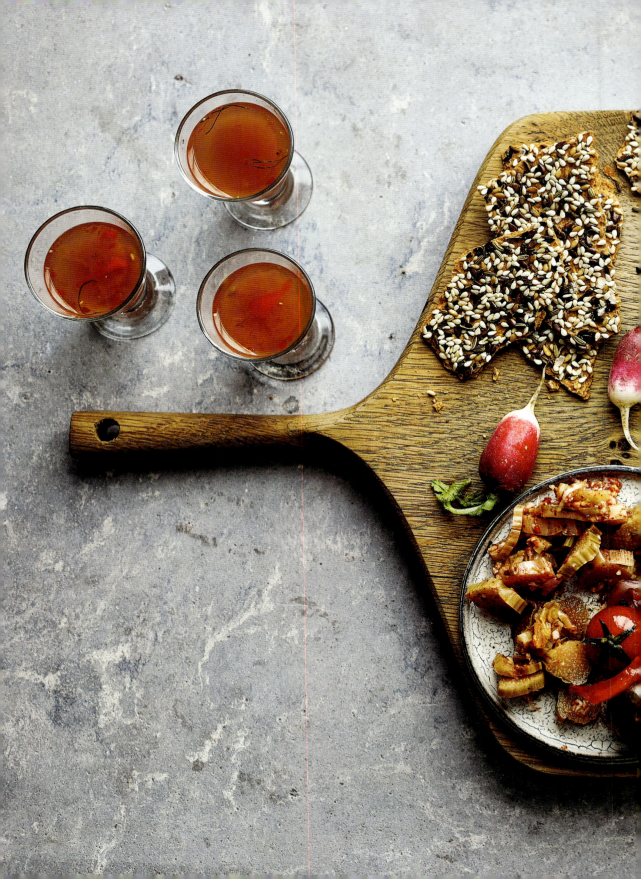

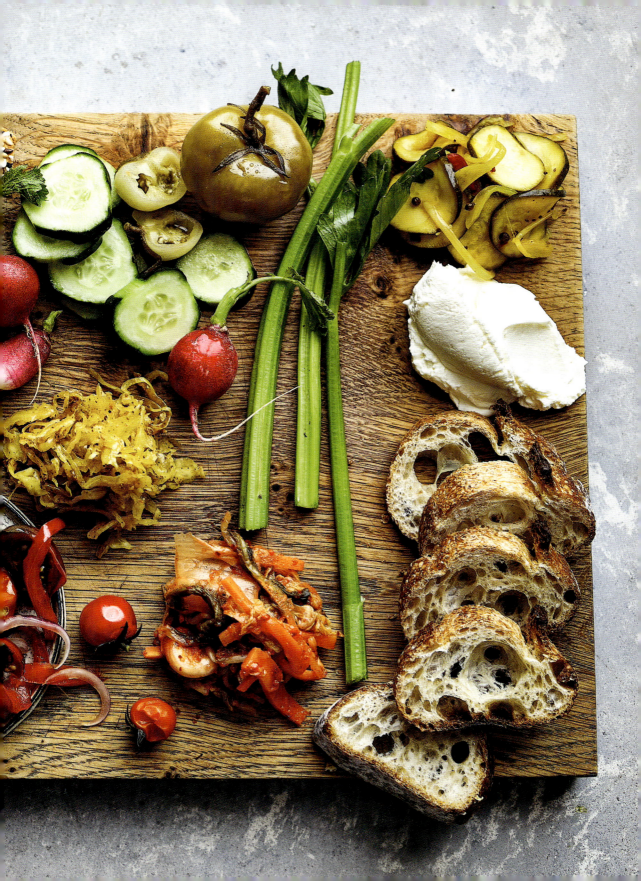

Sauercaccia

As someone who enjoys baking but is not a baker, I crave low-effort and high-reward recipes. This no-knead riff on a focaccia needs time to let the yeast work its magic, but as with a lot of baking, it's quite a relaxing and passive process, requiring only small bursts of active work. Not unlike fermenting vegetables.

The star of this bake is the sauerkraut topping. Older sauerkraut is best as it has a deeper fermented flavor. The sauercaccia uses a lot of sauerkraut, but through its density you get a spectrum of flavor and texture: The flavors intensify, the sauerkraut gets crispy on top and jammy underneath.

Any sauerkraut will work here but my favorites are the Garam Masala Sauerkraut (see page 36) and Chile, Orange & Coriander Sauerkraut (see page 47), which I have used in the accompanying image. They deliver on flavor and the latter is particularly stunning when it comes out of the oven. *See photo on the next page.*

PREP TIME: 30 MINUTES + 2 hours proving
COOK TIME: 30–40 MINUTES

Put the yeast in a small bowl with the sugar and 350ml (1¼ cups plus 3 tablespoons) lukewarm water and whisk together; set aside for 5 minutes until frothy, which shows that the yeast is ready to be used.

In a large bowl (or an electric mixer fitted with a dough hook), mix the flour and salt with the yeasty liquid until fully combined. If using an electric mixer at medium-high speed, this should take 5–7 minutes. It'll be a fairly sticky dough and should become stretchy. Scrape down the sides of the bowl and form the dough into a rough ball. Cover it with a teaspoon of extra virgin olive oil, using your hands to ensure there's a layer of oil all over the dough, then cover the bowl with a damp kitchen towel or plastic wrap, move it to a warm area of your kitchen, and leave the dough to rise for an hour, until doubled in size.

Pour 2 tablespoons of extra virgin olive oil onto the baking sheet, ensuring it's equally distributed, followed by a scattering of semolina: This will ensure the bread does not stick to the sheet.

Makes 12 squares

2¼ tsp instant yeast

1 tsp sugar

500g (3⅔ cups) high-protein bread flour

3 tsp salt

1 tsp extra virgin olive oil, plus 2 tbsp for oiling the tray, plus extra to drizzle

1 tbsp semolina

250g (1⅔ cups) sauerkraut, gently squeezed and drained

flaky sea salt and pepper

SPECIAL EQUIPMENT: 33 x 23-cm (13 x 9-in) baking sheet

Deflate the dough with a swift punch and scrape it onto the baking sheet. Using your fingers (and a bit of force), spread the dough out so it completely covers the tray, pushing it into the corners. Cover with a damp clean kitchen towel or plastic wrap and let rise for a further hour.

Preheat the oven to 450°F (230°C).

Sprinkle the sauerkraut over the dough. Use your fingers to press the sauerkraut into the dough while continuing to spread the dough out over the baking sheet. It may seem like a lot of sauerkraut, so take the time to ensure it's evenly distributed both on top and throughout the dough. Drizzle with a little extra virgin olive oil and season generously with sea salt and pepper.

Bake for 30–40 minutes or until the sides of the bread have released from the tray, the bread is golden, and the sauerkraut is slightly charred and crispy. Leave to cool to room temperature before cutting into squares and serving. The bread can be easily reheated in the oven.

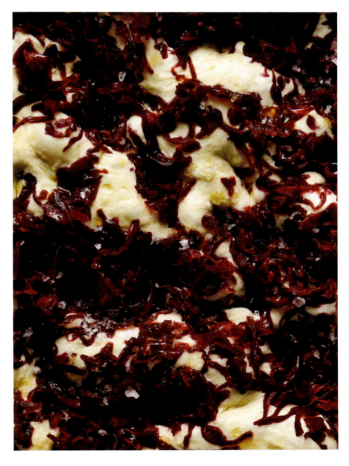

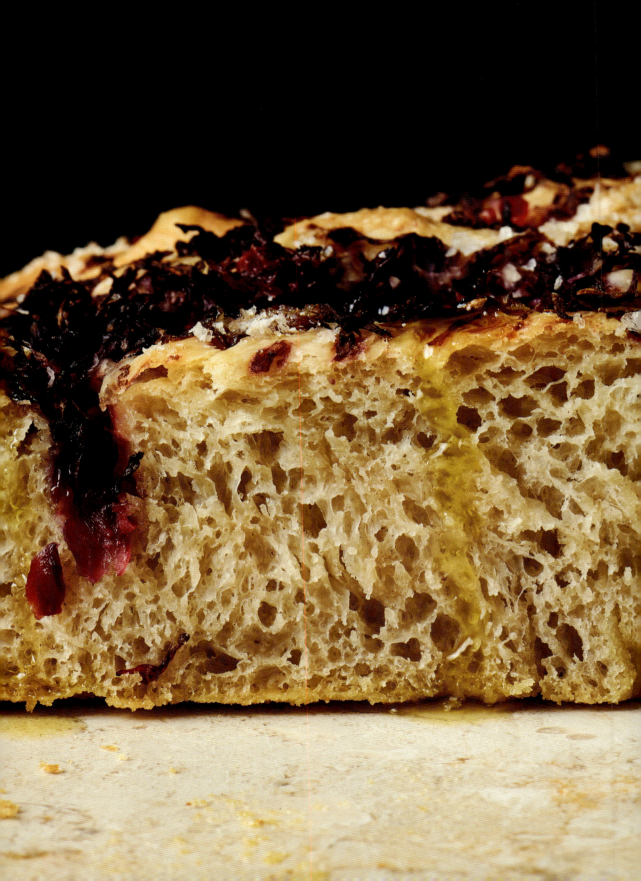

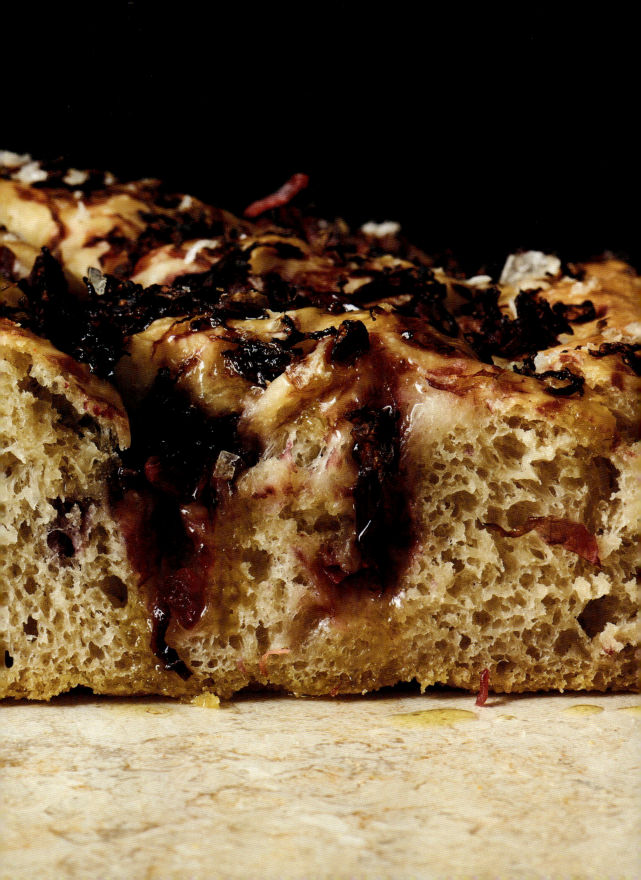

Sauerkraut Latkes with Dill Yogurt

I grew up in a culturally Jewish community in Chicago and was exposed to Ashkenazi Jewish cuisine at a young age. A lot of the recipes and traditions inevitably seeped into my family's cooking and it became a tradition in my home to make latkes over the holiday period. This cultural culinary connection ran deep. Little known fun fact: I co-led the Jewish cooking club at my college.

Latkes are such a crowd pleaser and are something I make pretty much every year in December when we're having friends over for a festive meal. They're excellent as a starter, and can be elevated if served with fish roe or smoked salmon. They're also quite the special brunch item.

The addition of sauerkraut makes the latkes a bit lighter and more complex in flavor: It seems like an obvious combination given sauerkraut's ubiquity in Eastern Europe. All of the sauerkraut varieties in this book will work well here, but be sure to really squeeze all residual brine out of the sauerkraut (and the water from the grated potatoes).

PREP TIME: 20 MINUTES | COOK TIME: 20–25 MINUTES

Using a box grater, or a food processor with the grater attachment, grate the potatoes and onion. It may feel odd to grate an onion using a box grater but do it gently and use the outer onion layer as a sort of protection as you grate. Mix the grated potato and onion together in a bowl and leave for a few minutes, then squeeze out as much liquid as possible from the mixture. You can do this with a clean kitchen towel; doing it diligently with your bare hands works as well. Minimizing the water is very important: You do not want the potato mixture to be too wet before frying. Discard the liquid.

Add the drained sauerkraut to the potato mixture, then add the flour, cornstarch, eggs, and salt, and season with pepper. Mix thoroughly.

Make the dill yogurt by mixing all of the ingredients together.

Heat a large frying pan over a medium-high heat and add enough oil to shallow fry (about 5mm/¼in). To check that the oil is hot enough, drop in a small amount of the latke mixture: If it immediately starts to crisp and bubble, you're good to go! Line a tray with paper towels.

Use 2 tablespoons to measure out the latke mixture. Flatten it in your hands (gently!) and carefully drop it into the hot oil using a metal spatula.

Continue adding latkes quickly and carefully as the latke mixture will get watery as it sits, but do not overcrowd the pan, as too many latkes will lower the temperature of the oil.

Cook each latke for 3–4 minutes on each side, and flip when you see the edges browning; if the latke is ready it should release from the pan and will be golden brown. Drain the latkes on the lined tray and season with flaky sea salt while still hot.

If making larger batches, preheat the oven to 400°F (200°C) and keep the latkes in the oven as you finish frying them.

Serve immediately with the dill yogurt, or make a more festive dish with fish roe, smoked salmon, capers, and additional sauerkraut, if using. Once cooled, the latkes can be frozen.

Makes 10 latkes

250g (9oz) white potatoes, peeled

1 onion, peeled

250g (1⅔ cups) sauerkraut, squeezed and drained

1 tbsp all-purpose flour

1 tbsp cornstarch

2 medium eggs

½ tsp flaky sea salt, plus extra for seasoning

black pepper

vegetable oil for shallow frying

FOR THE DILL YOGURT

150g (⅔ cup) full-fat yogurt

1 tbsp lemon juice

handful of fresh dill, roughly chopped

TO SERVE (OPTIONAL)

fish roe

smoked salmon

capers

sauerkraut

SPECIAL EQUIPMENT: food processor (optional)

STARTERS

Fermented Gazpacho

Do you ever think about what would be on your dream dinner party menu? In many of my scribbled plans, I return to this dish. It's familiar, bright, and complex, and would be served as a canapé—in shot glasses—since all dream dinner parties start with canapés. This is such a summery dish and as it's so fresh (despite the fermented elements), you definitely want to go for the best quality ingredients you can find—this is true for the tomatoes as well as the extra virgin olive oil.

And lastly, do yourself a favor and keep all of the leftover brine in a new (and smaller) jar. This brine could be used to kickstart a new ferment to add a strong tomato essence in other recipes: I've been using it in salad dressings, and a martini is calling its name (see Tomatini, page 260).

PREP TIME: 15 MINUTES

Strain the vegetables from the fermented tomatoes, reserving the fermented brine. Put the strained vegetables and cucumber into a food processor or blender and blitz to your desired consistency. I prefer it slightly chunky.

Add the olive oil, white wine vinegar, and 60–80ml (¼–⅓ cup) of the reserved brine (the smaller quantity will make a thicker gazpacho), give it a good stir, season with salt and pepper if needed, and serve.

For a really cold gazpacho, transfer it to the fridge for an hour or add a few ice cubes to each bowl.

Garnish with fresh dill, diced cucumber, and a healthy glug of extra virgin olive oil. This can be kept in an airtight container in the fridge for 2–3 days.

Serves 2–3

- 1 recipe of Gazpacho Cherry Tomatoes (see page 43)
- 1 cucumber, about 200g (7oz), peeled and cut into 5-cm (2-in) chunks
- 60ml (¼ cup) extra virgin olive oil
- 1 tbsp white wine vinegar
- salt and pepper

TO SERVE

fresh dill
diced cucumber
extra virgin olive oil

SPECIAL EQUIPMENT: food processor or blender

Pickled Fruit Tart with Goat Cheese

I love a cheese platter as much as the next person but I tend to judge it on what else is included: not just a variety of crackers but, most importantly, the chutneys and pickles which are a necessary foil to the richness of cheese. Pickled fruit works amazingly on this cheesy puff pastry tart, slightly caramelized and nearly bursting against a creamy base of goat cheese and mascarpone. It's further elevated with a drizzle of honey and pink peppercorns. For a fairly easy recipe, this gives an elegant brunch vibe (or even meal prep as the leftovers are delicious cold), served alongside a nice salad.

I'm all about the crust-to-cheese ratio, so I usually make this as two smaller tarts from a standard pack of ready-made puff pastry. But there's nothing stopping you from making a massive one! *See photos on the next page.*

PREP TIME: 30 MINUTES | COOK TIME: 30–35 MINUTES

Preheat the oven to 400°F (200°C). Transfer a baking sheet to the oven to warm up while you prepare the tart (around 10 minutes).

Mix the mascarpone and goat cheese with the pickle brine in a bowl. Move it to the fridge while you prepare the fruit and puff pastry.

Unroll the puff pastry, keeping it on its provided parchment paper. Cut the puff pastry in half crosswise, making two rectangles. Using a knife, gently score a 2-cm (¾-in) border around each rectangle and then, using a fork, prick the pastry inside the border.

Smear half of the cheese mixture over each tart, within the border. Add the pieces of pickled fruit. Sprinkle with small sprigs of fresh thyme and pink peppercorns and then lightly brush the pastry borders with beaten egg.

Transfer the tarts and parchment paper onto the preheated baking sheet and bake for 30–35 minutes until cooked through and golden.

Drizzle with honey and sprinkle with fresh thyme leaves and serve once cooled to room temperature.

Serves 6

125g (½ cup) mascarpone
250g (⅔ cup) soft goat cheese
3 tbsp pickle brine
12–15 pieces of Pickled Fruit (see page 120–121, use a variety), cut into similar-size pieces
One 320-g (11-oz) pack ready-rolled puff pastry (if frozen, defrost completely)
a few sprigs of fresh thyme (keep a few leaves to garnish)
1 tsp pink peppercorns, roughly crushed with a mortar and pestle
1 egg, beaten
clear honey

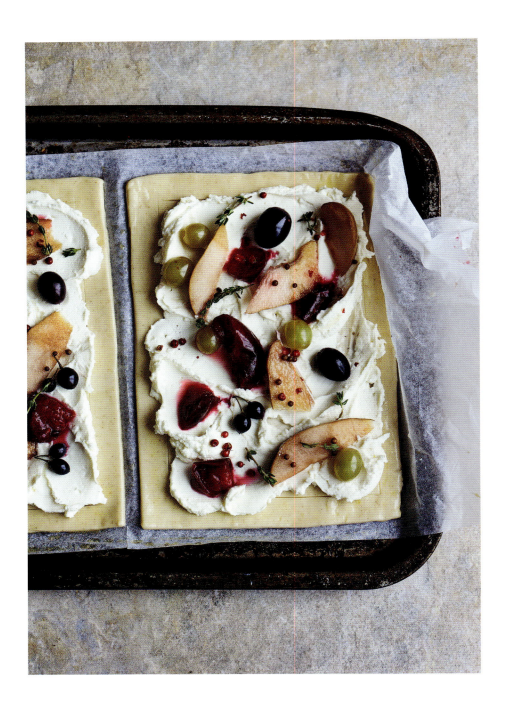

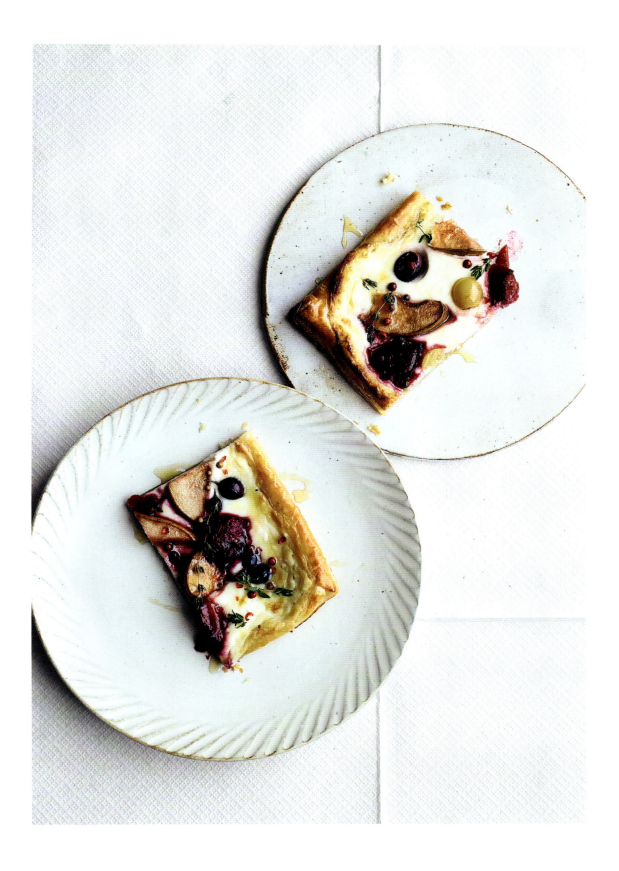

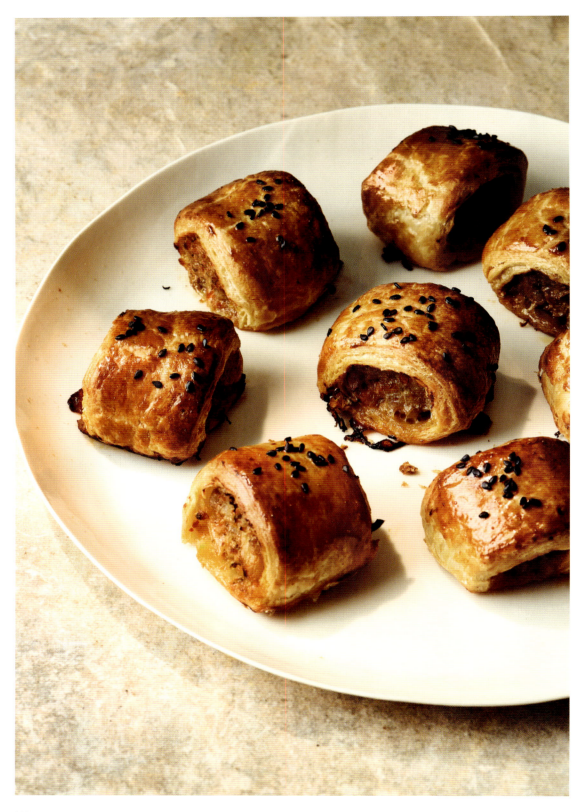

Kimchi & Fennel Sausage Rolls

One of the first "British" food items I made for my family back in the States were sausage rolls and they were a roaring success. They've now become a mainstay in our home—and are the perfect finger food for all of those festive gatherings. That said, we've been guilty of polishing off a full batch of these just between the two of us.

The combination of kimchi and fennel seeds is my twist on the fennel-forward Italian sausages I grew up on in Chicago. It is a great way to use up older kimchi that you may not want to eat fresh—don't let all of that heat and complex flavor go to waste.

PREP TIME: 30 MINUTES + 30 minutes chilling
COOK TIME: 20–25 MINUTES

Heat a frying pan over a medium-high heat, add the oil, and stir-fry the chopped kimchi with the sugar until jammy and all of the liquid has evaporated, around 5–7 minutes. Remove from the heat.
  Grind 1 tablespoon of the fennel seeds in a mortar and pestle or spice grinder, leaving the rest whole.
  In a mixing bowl, combine the sausage meat, ground and whole fennel seeds, and the cooked kimchi. Mix thoroughly and leave in the fridge for at least 30 minutes for the flavors to meld.
  Preheat the oven to 450°F (230°C). Line a baking sheet with parchment paper. Cut the puff pastry in half lengthwise.
  Divide the sausage-kimchi mixture in half and roll each piece into a compact long sausage the same length as the pastry. Place the sausage-kimchi mixture on the pastry, about two-thirds of the way in.
  Brush one long side of the pastry with beaten egg, then roll the pastry tightly around the sausage-kimchi mixture, finishing with the seam side underneath. Repeat with the other piece of pastry.
  Using a sharp knife, cut the two long sausage rolls each into six 5-cm (2-in) segments, brush with beaten egg, and then sprinkle with black sesame seeds.
  Put the sausage rolls onto the lined baking sheet, spaced apart as they will expand slightly as they cook. Bake for 15–20 minutes until golden brown.
  Once cooled, the sausage rolls can be frozen.

Makes 12 sausage rolls

1 tsp vegetable oil
300g (2 cups) kimchi, chopped
1½ tsp sugar
1 tbsp plus 1½ tsp fennel seeds
500g (1lb 2oz) sausage meat
One 320-g (11-oz) pack ready-rolled puff pastry (if frozen, defrost completely)
2 eggs, beaten
black sesame seeds

Kimchi Onion Bhajis with Cilantro & Mint Miso Chutney

This recipe encapsulates so much of what I love about cooking: bringing together delicious flavors from across the world. When I first moved to the UK, onion bhajis became an obsession (alongside Scotch eggs, but that's for another time). As a self-proclaimed fritter lover, they left an immediate impression. As with many new beginnings, this discovery coincided with another realization. It wasn't easy to find kimchi—something that I had taken for granted back in the States—which kickstarted my monthly kimchi making. This recipe is therefore a celebration of my move to the UK, grounding myself in routine, yet launching me into new and creative directions.

The trick with this dish is using old (and very fermented) kimchi, as this equals flavor. The microbes won't survive the heat, but the kimchi will add complex umami while balancing the earthiness of the chickpea flour. Don't have kimchi? Try another over-fermented pickle, such as sauerkraut.

The bhajis come together quickly, so they can be easily made as you chat with friends in the kitchen. You will also probably gain brownie points for deep-frying. They're delicious as they are (thanks to the kimchi!) but really pop with vibrancy when paired with the zingy cilantro and mint miso chutney. The chutney is also delicious slathered on your favorite sandwich, but truth be told, you'll probably get through most of it with these bhajis. *See photos on the next page.*

PREP TIME: 20 MINUTES | COOK TIME: 15 MINUTES

Prepare the chutney by roughly chopping the herbs, including stems and leaves (unless the mint stems are particularly woody, in which case compost them), and adding them to a food processor, along with the peanuts, miso, lemon zest and juice, honey, salt, and turmeric. Blitz to make a fairly chunky chutney.

To get a dipping consistency, add 3 tablespoons of water and the yogurt and blitz again. You may want to adjust the salt to taste, but be aware that miso is salty.

Transfer the chutney to the fridge while you make the bhajis. It will keep in the fridge for several days and can be made ahead of time.

To make the bhajis, fill a deep cast-iron pan or wok with vegetable oil (no more than one-third full for safety) and turn the heat to high. If you're using a deep-fat fryer, heat the oil to 350°F (180°C).

While the oil is warming up, prepare the bhaji mixture. Mix the onion, garlic, and kimchi in a large bowl. Add the chickpea flour, turmeric, and salt and mix well. Add about 160ml (⅔ cup) of water and stir to make a slightly loose batter.

To check that the oil is hot enough, drop a very small amount of batter into the oil: If it immediately starts to float and sizzle, it's ready.

Line a tray with paper towels. Gently drop generous tablespoons of the batter into the oil and cook for around 90 seconds on each side. Do not overcrowd the pan, as too many bhajis will lower the temperature of the oil. You'll know they're ready to flip when they rise up from the bottom of the pan. When both sides are golden brown, drain them on the lined tray to absorb excess oil and immediately sprinkle with salt.

You can freeze any leftover bhajis: They reheat wonderfully in the oven.

Makes approximately 14 bhajis

FOR THE CILANTRO & MINT MISO CHUTNEY

50g (3 cups) fresh cilantro

50g (3 cups) fresh mint

60g (¼ cup plus 2 tbsp) peanuts, unsalted and unroasted, roughly chopped

1 tbsp plus 1½ tsp red miso

zest of 1 lemon and 60ml (¼ cup) lemon juice

2 tsp clear honey

¼ tsp salt

¼ tsp ground turmeric

60g (¼ cup) full-fat yogurt

FOR THE KIMCHI BHAJIS

vegetable oil for deep-frying

1 white onion, peeled and finely sliced

2 garlic cloves, peeled and finely chopped

250g (1⅔ cups) kimchi, roughly chopped

165g (1¾ cups) chickpea flour

1 tsp ground turmeric

1 tsp salt, plus extra for seasoning

SPECIAL EQUIPMENT: deep-fat fryer (optional); food processor (for the chutney)

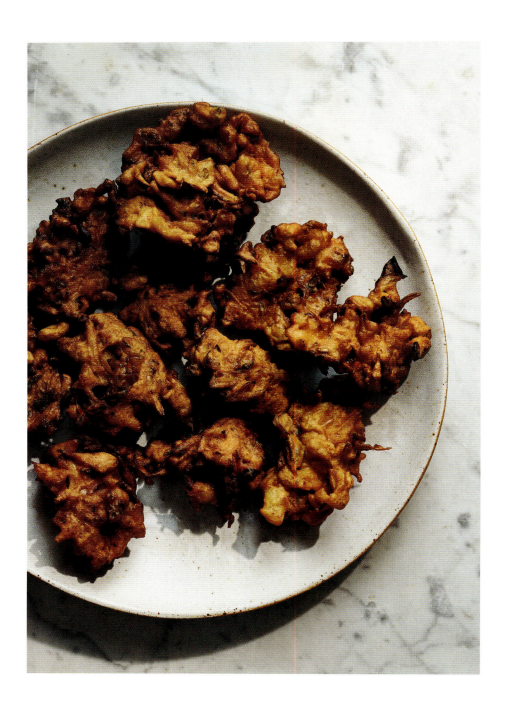

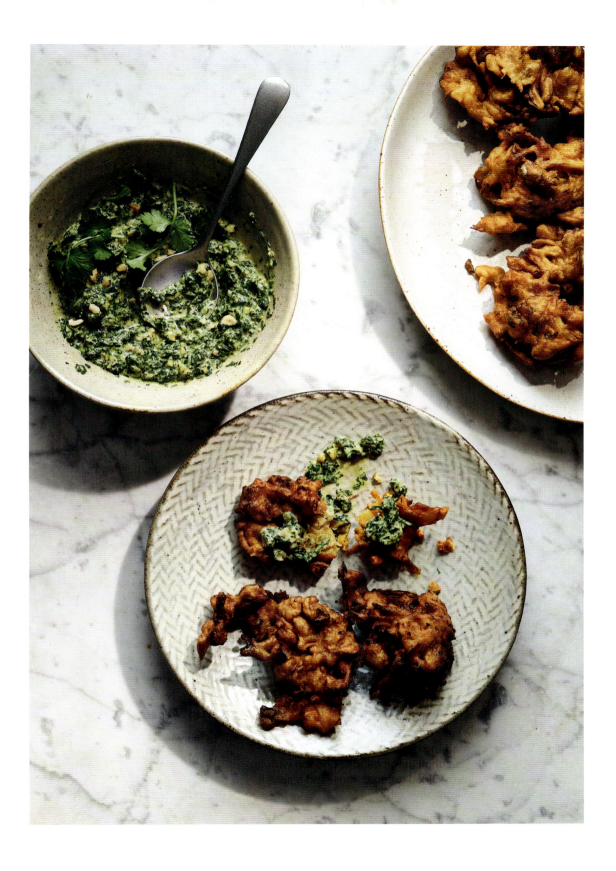

Miso Hummus with Umami Zucchini & Pine Nuts

Miso and beans are a match made in heaven. While I have nothing against more traditional hummus recipes, there's something incredibly comforting about a miso hummus. I suppose that's the power of umami, which is here amplified by the zucchini topping: thin pieces, fried until brown and cooked in a sweet and savory glaze. This hummus leans a bit Japanese, but with the ubiquity of miso in modern cooking it can easily accompany other cuisines: alongside a Middle Eastern feast, with your next barbecue spread, or as an excellent starter ahead of the Nasu Dengaku Moussaka (see page 228).

PREP TIME: 10 MINUTES | COOK TIME: 20 MINUTES

Put all of the hummus ingredients into a food processor and blitz to your preferred consistency. I like very smooth hummus, which the ice facilitates. Season with salt, if needed, but note that the red miso is salty, as will be the zucchini topping.

To make the zucchini topping, start by toasting the pine nuts in a dry frying pan over a low heat for 3–5 minutes, until lightly browned and nutty. Stir them occasionally and keep a watchful eye as it's very easy to over-toast and burn them. Transfer the nuts to a small bowl.

Slice the zucchini into 5-mm (¼-in) rounds and place them in a mixing bowl. Add the olive oil and mix to ensure all of the slices are coated in oil. Put the frying pan over a medium-high heat and fry the zucchini slices for 2–3 minutes on each side until browned: Cook in batches, being mindful not to overcrowd the pan. Drain on paper towels. When you've cooked all of the zucchini, use a piece of paper towel to wipe out any residual oil from the pan.

Put the zucchini back into the pan and reduce the heat to low. Mix the mirin, miso, and red pepper flakes in a small bowl and then add to the pan. The mixture should reduce very quickly.

To serve, spread the hummus in a shallow bowl or plate, add the zucchini in the middle, and top with the toasted pine nuts, sliced green onions, and a splash of good extra virgin olive oil.

Serves 4–6

FOR THE HUMMUS

500g (3 cups) cooked lima beans (rinsed and drained from two 400-g/14-oz cans), or canned chickpeas

3 tbsp tahini

2 tbsp red miso

zest of 1 lemon and 2 tbsp lemon juice

100ml (¼ cup plus 3 tbsp) olive oil

handful of ice (4–5 cubes)

FOR THE ZUCCHINI TOPPING

1 tbsp pine nuts

1 zucchini, about 350g (12oz)

3 tbsp olive oil

1 tbsp mirin

1 tsp red or white miso

¼ tsp red pepper flakes

TO SERVE

1–2 green onions, trimmed and thinly sliced

extra virgin olive oil

SPECIAL EQUIPMENT: food processor

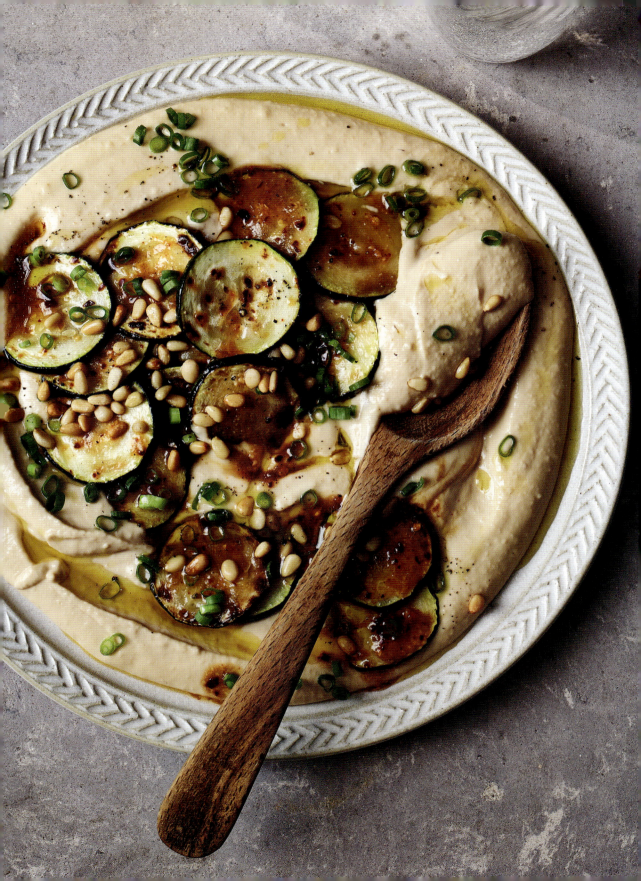

Kimchi Fried Rice Comté Arancini

Sounds glorious, right? I would say that this is your answer to using up leftover kimchi fried rice, but when does that ever happen? So let this be the call to action to make a batch specifically for this! Using fried rice is a faster process than risotto-based arancini—in both the cooking and cooling. And the flavors here work so well together—savory sweet gochujang-laced, tangy kimchi fried rice and sesame oil amplified by the nuttiness of Comté cheese. Mozzarella can work here (and will increase the likelihood of that ultimate cheese pull); however, Comté is a special cheese and it truly shines in this dish.

This recipe may seem like a lot of work but it's well worth the effort. It can easily be scaled up (which I generally recommend when deep-frying) to feed a crowd. *See photos on the next pages.*

PREP TIME: 20 MINUTES + 30 minutes chilling
COOK TIME: 25–35 MINUTES

Heat a frying pan over a medium heat with 1 tablespoon of oil and stir-fry the kimchi for 2–3 minutes. Add the cooked and cooled rice, followed by the kimchi brine and gochujang. Stir-fry for 5–10 minutes, until combined, with each grain of rice a bright red. Add the sesame oil and sesame seeds, mix it all together, then decant into a bowl to cool.

While the fried rice cools, prepare the arancini assembly line: Put the cheese, bread crumbs, flour, and eggs into four separate shallow bowls.

Divide the fried rice into eight equal amounts and, using your hands, roll them into balls and insert about 1 tablespoon of the grated cheese into the center. Pinch and shape the ball to ensure there's an even layer of rice surrounding the cheese. Repeat with the remaining fried rice and cheese. Put the balls in the fridge for 30 minutes to firm up. Line a baking sheet with parchment paper.

To deep-fry: First dredge the arancini in the flour, then coat them in the egg (letting excess egg drip back into the bowl), and then put them into the bowl of bread crumbs, pressing the crumbs on to ensure each arancini is entirely coated and holding together

Serves 8 (one arancino per person)

1 tbsp vegetable oil, plus extra for deep-frying

200g (1⅓ cups) kimchi, chopped

400g (2½ cups) jasmine rice, cooked and cooled

60–120ml (¼–½ cup) kimchi brine, topped up with water if needed to make a total of 120ml (½ cup)

2 tbsp gochujang

1 tbsp toasted sesame oil

1 tbsp sesame seeds

100g (½ cup) Comté cheese, grated

170g (2 cups) panko bread crumbs

120g (1 cup) all-purpose flour

2 eggs, beaten

salt and pepper

SPECIAL EQUIPMENT: deep-fat fryer (optional)

well. Put the arancini onto the lined baking sheet and return them to the fridge while you heat the oil.

Fill a deep cast-iron pan or wok with vegetable oil (no more than one-third full for safety) and turn the heat to high. If you're using a deep-fat fryer, heat the oil to 350°F (180°C). To check that the oil is hot enough, drop a very small amount of the panko into the oil: If it immediately starts to float and sizzle, it's ready to start frying. Line a tray with paper towels.

Fry the arancini for 6–8 minutes, in batches if necessary; don't overcrowd the pan. Flip them after 3–4 minutes to ensure they are crisp all over. Transfer them to the prepared tray to drain the excess oil and season them with salt and pepper. Serve immediately, or cool and freeze.

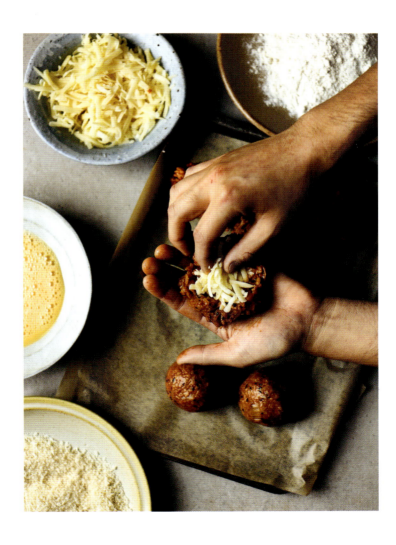

STARTERS

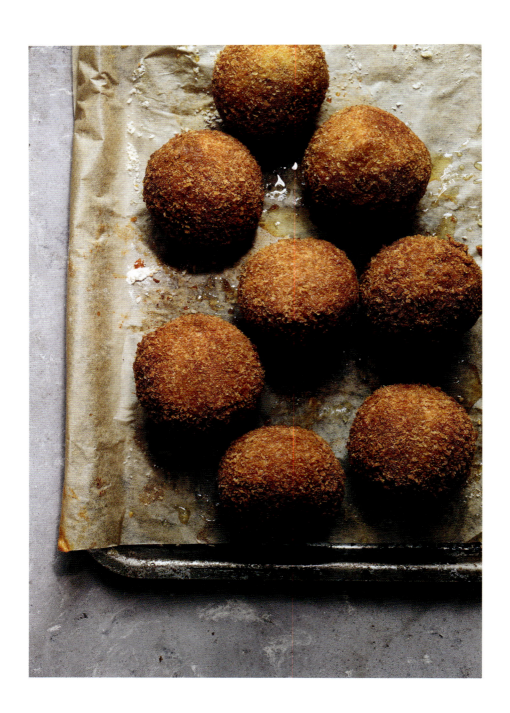

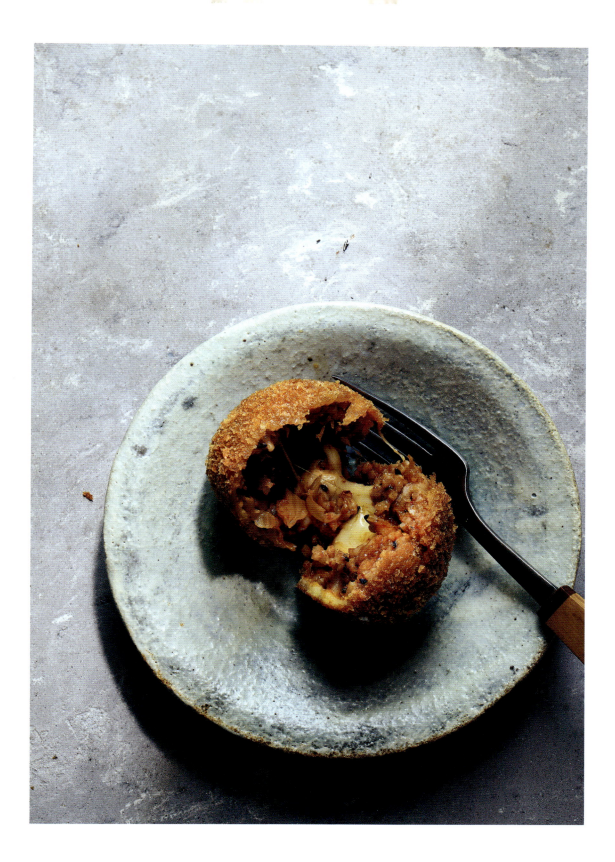

Miso Butter Corn Ribs Elote

The current trend for small and sharing plates is a beautiful thing: a focus on ease of eating when spending time with friends and family. I've often found corn a challenging ingredient in these settings—I'm a fan of eating with my hands, but it can sometimes be difficult and messy. Enter corn ribs. Only requiring a sharp knife and a bit of strength, cutting corn on the cob into quarters lengthwise increases the surface area, leading to more flavor from the marinade and more crispiness as it bakes in the oven. But if you're feeling lazy and making this for two people, you can use one cob per person and leave them whole.

This dish brings together two of my favorite styles of corn on the cob: miso butter corn, a nod to childhood memories from trips to Japan; and the Mexican elote I ate in the Pilsen neighborhood of Chicago as a teenager. I'd recommend doubling the recipe as, in my experience, people like seconds!

PREP TIME: 15 MINUTES | COOK TIME: 45 MINUTES

Preheat the oven to 400°F (200°C). Line a baking sheet with parchment paper.

Cut the corn into ribs by cutting each cob into quarters lengthwise. Hold the corn cob vertically and carefully use a sharp knife and a rocking motion to cut downward. Once you have the initial cut, it's easy to slice through, but please take care.

In a small saucepan, heat all of the ingredients for the miso butter sauce until everything is combined and starts to bubble. Remove from the heat.

Put the corn ribs in a bowl, add the miso butter sauce, and stir to coat evenly. Transfer the corn ribs to the prepared baking sheet.

Bake the corn ribs for 35 minutes, turning them halfway through and basting them with any leftover sauce. If you want them to be crispier, keep them in the oven for a further 5–7 minutes.

Arrange the corn ribs on a plate and garnish with crumbled feta, chopped cilantro, and the juice of half a lime. Cut the other lime half into quarters and serve with the corn ribs.

Sprinkle with chile flakes of your choice. This is also good with Quick-Pickled Red Onions (see page 114) and Quick-Pickled Kombucha Chiles (see page 112).

Serves 4 (two ribs per person)

- 2 ears of corn
- 3 tbsp feta, crumbled
- 25g (1oz) fresh cilantro, stems and leaves finely chopped
- 1 lime, halved
- chile flakes for color and mild heat, such as Aleppo, ancho, or Kashmiri; I recommend Tajin Mexican-style seasoning if you can get it; or try Kimchi Sprinkles (see page 76)

FOR THE MISO BUTTER SAUCE

- 3 tbsp miso
- 4 tbsp unsalted butter, at room temperature
- 1 tbsp honey
- 2 tsp soy sauce, preferably Japanese or light soy

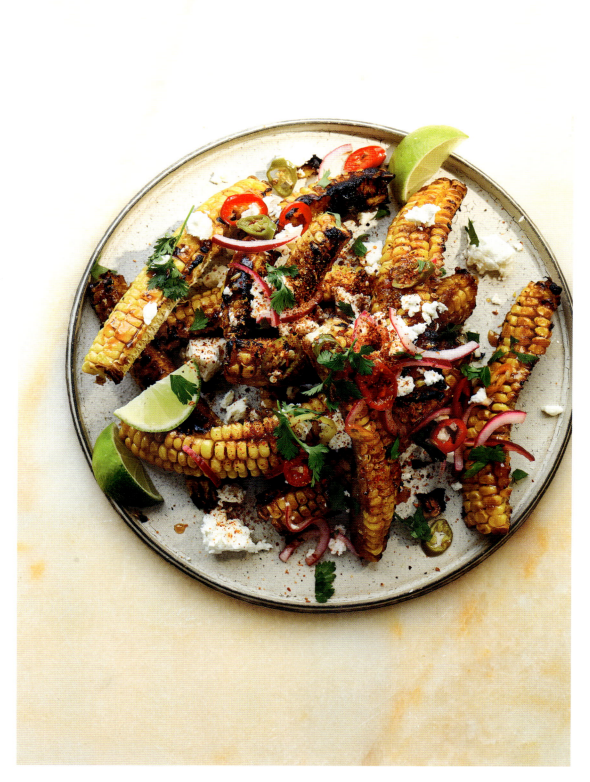

Kimchi & Cheddar Biscuits

These savory and flaky biscuits, packed with cheese and kimchi, are my definition of the perfect snack. Fresh from the oven, slathered with butter, and then topped with a dollop of Red Onion & Kimchi Chutney (see opposite), they truly hold their own in terms of flavor. Bring them to a family gathering, brunch, or picnic, or enjoy them alongside a soup or salad. They are best eaten warm, however, so if you can, re-warm them in the oven for the full experience. *See photo on the next page.*

PREP TIME: 30 MINUTES | COOK TIME: 15 MINUTES

Makes 12 small biscuits

- 210g (1⅔ cups) all-purpose flour, plus extra for dusting
- 1 tbsp baking powder
- ½ tsp baking soda
- 1 tsp salt
- 113g (8 tbsp) cold unsalted butter
- 80g (⅔ cup) cheddar, grated
- 100g (¾ cup) kimchi, chopped
- 150ml (½ cup plus 2 tbsp) whole milk
- 1 medium egg, beaten

Preheat the oven to 450°F (230°C). Line a baking sheet with parchment paper.

In a mixing bowl, combine the flour, baking powder, baking soda, and salt. Using a box grater, grate in the butter. If you do not have a box grater, cut the butter into small cubes and use your fingers to crumble the butter into the dry ingredients until the mixture has a rough bread-crumb consistency. Do not over-handle the butter as it needs to stay relatively cool as you make the dough.

Add the cheese and chopped kimchi and start adding milk as you knead it into a rough dough. Use slightly less or more milk if needed—the dough should still be slightly crumbly and not too wet.

On a flour-dusted surface, roll out the dough to a rectangle, about 20 x 15cm (8 x 6in). Fold this in half and roll it out again. Repeat the folding and rolling once more for a total of two times, working quickly to ensure the butter does not melt too much. This will give the biscuits ample buttery flakiness.

Roll out the dough to a rectangle about 2cm (¾in) thick. Cut into 6 squares and then cut each piece in half to make 12 small biscuits.

Arrange the biscuits on the lined baking sheet and brush with beaten egg for a beautiful glaze. Bake for 12–15 minutes until golden brown. Move to a wire rack to cool slightly before serving.

Once cooled, these can be frozen.

Red Onion & Kimchi Chutney, Two Ways

I developed two chutney recipes, expecting that one would reign supreme, but my friends liked both of them. The only difference is the form of acidity used to deglaze and flavor the chutney. Red wine vinegar works well, and is more reminiscent of the traditional red onion chutneys you may be familiar with, but if you have enough kimchi brine, try it out for a spicier twist on this chutney. View this as a fun reminder that different forms of acidity can and should be swapped around in your home cooking.

This makes a sizable batch of chutney, so it's a perfect excuse to use up your small jars and gift them to friends and family! *See photo on the next page.*

PREP TIME: 15 MINUTES | COOK TIME: 25–30 MINUTES

Heat a heavy-bottomed pan over a medium-low heat, then add the olive oil, red onion, and chopped kimchi. Cook for 15 minutes, until caramelized and jammy. The volume will decrease considerably.

Add the sugar, fish sauce, and red wine vinegar (or kimchi brine), and continue cooking for 10–15 minutes until the liquid has reduced, leaving a thick and glossy chutney. Let this cool to room temperature before consuming.

The chutney will keep for 3 months in the fridge.

Makes one 500-ml (1-pint) jar (or decant into smaller jars)

- 2 tbsp olive oil
- 400g (14oz) red onion, peeled and thinly sliced
- 300g (2 cups) kimchi, chopped
- 150g (¾ cup) brown sugar
- 1 tsp fish sauce
- 200ml (¾ cup plus 1 tbsp) red wine vinegar or kimchi brine

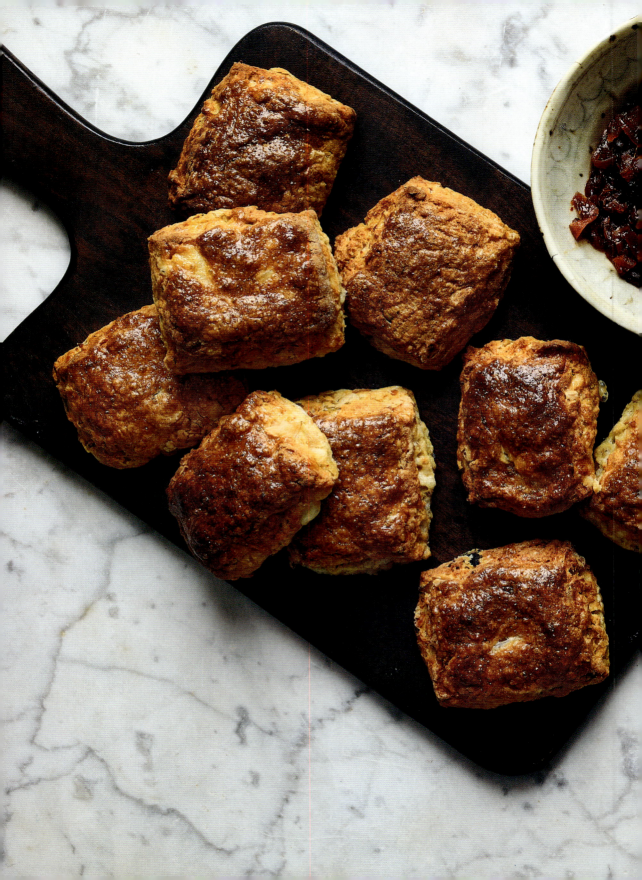

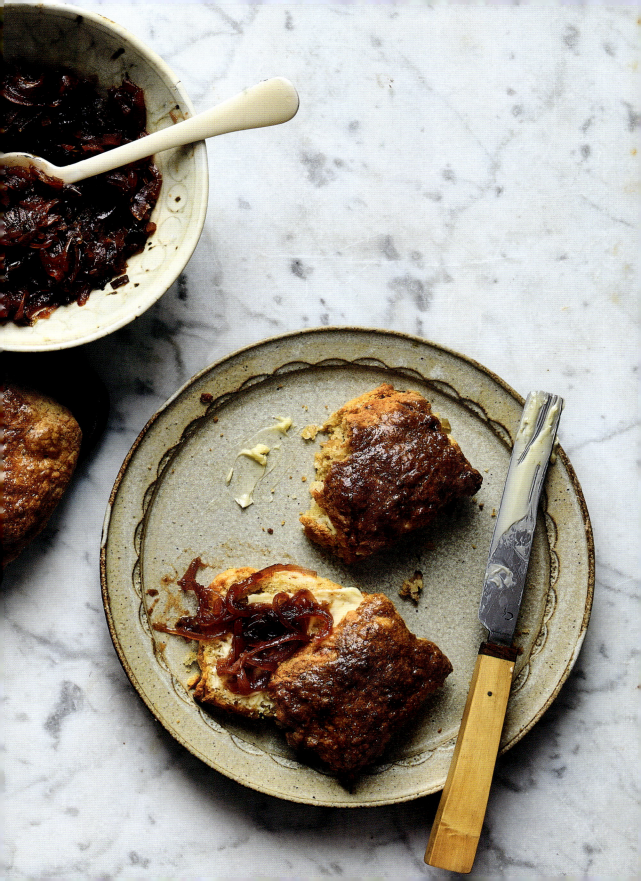

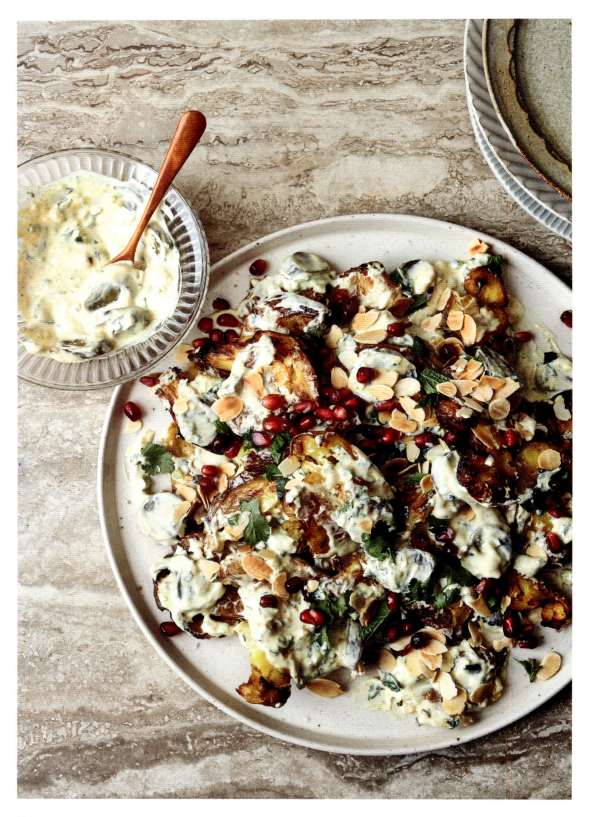

Curried Pickle Smashed Potato Salad

Trendy smashed roasted potatoes meet their match in juicy dill pickles, fresh herbs, and tangy pickled red onions against the backdrop of a creamy curried dressing, all topped with pomegranate and toasted flaked almonds. For what looks like a lot of effort, this recipe is simple and quick to assemble. It is great at room temperature so it's a perfect dish for entertaining, and all elements can be made ahead. Once the potatoes are dressed, however, I think it's best eaten the same day. Plating the salad in a shallow layer means that every bite has all of the requisite textures and flavors.

PREP TIME: 15 MINUTES | COOK TIME: 50-55 MINUTES

Boil the potatoes in water, with 1 tablespoon of salt, for around 15 minutes or until fork tender. Drain the potatoes and put them back in the pan to let them steam dry.

Preheat the oven to 450°F (230°C). Line a baking sheet with parchment paper.

Drizzle 2 tablespoons of the oil over the potatoes and toss so the oil is evenly distributed.

Put the potatoes on the lined baking sheet, spacing them apart, and use the bottom of a glass jar to smash them until they're about 5mm (¼in) thick. Brush the remaining tablespoon of oil over the smashed potatoes and roast for 35-40 minutes until golden brown.

While the potatoes are roasting, make the dressing by combining all of the ingredients in a bowl or jar. Season with salt and pepper if needed, but note that the potatoes will also be salted.

Once the potatoes are done, season liberally with salt and pepper. Let them cool for a few minutes and then toss them with the dressing.

Assemble the salad on a large shallow plate: first the dressed potatoes, followed by the mint and cilantro leaves, toasted flaked almonds, and pomegranate seeds.

Serves 4-6

750g (1lb 10oz) baby potatoes

1 tbsp salt, plus extra for seasoning

3 tbsp vegetable oil

black pepper

20g (¼ cup) flaked almonds, lightly toasted, to garnish

pomegranate seeds to garnish

FOR THE DRESSING

125g (½ cup) full-fat yogurt

1 tbsp plus 1½ tsp mango chutney

½ tsp medium curry powder

100g (3.5oz) Sour Dill Pickles (see page 44), chopped into bite-size pieces

1 tbsp Sour Dill Pickle brine

2 green onions, trimmed and thinly sliced (greens and whites)

1 tbsp chopped fresh cilantro, plus extra leaves to garnish

1 tsp chopped fresh mint, plus extra leaves to garnish

10g (0.33oz) Quick-Pickled Red Onions (see page 114), finely chopped

Bitter Greens Salad with Pickled Pear Vinaigrette

Bitter greens—stronger flavored and generally more robust than other lettuce varieties—are my favorite ingredient for salads. Their flavor lends them well to an interesting salad, especially when you throw in praline pecans for sweetness and crunch and a punchy pickled pear vinaigrette. Feel free to use other pickled fruits—the other recipes in this book will all work with this vinaigrette.

PREP TIME: 10 MINUTES

Wash and dry the greens and put them into a serving bowl, along with the chopped parsley.

To make the vinaigrette, put all of the ingredients into a food processor and blitz until you have a chunky purée. Taste and adjust the seasoning. You can also make the dressing by hand: Finely chop the pickled fruit and whisk all of the ingredients together.

Add the dressing to the greens and parsley and toss. Sprinkle with the nuts and enjoy.

Serves 2–4

- 200–250g (7–9oz) mixed bitter greens, such as arugula, watercress, endive, and radicchio
- 50g (¾ cup) fresh parsley, roughly chopped
- handful of Miso Praline Sesame Pecans (see page 236), or alternatively your favorite sweet roasted nuts or similar crunchy element

FOR THE VINAIGRETTE

- approximately 60g (2oz) Pickled Pears (see page 121)
- 1 tbsp Pickled Pear brine
- 1 tsp Dijon mustard
- 2 tbsp extra virgin olive oil
- salt and pepper

SPECIAL EQUIPMENT: food processor (optional)

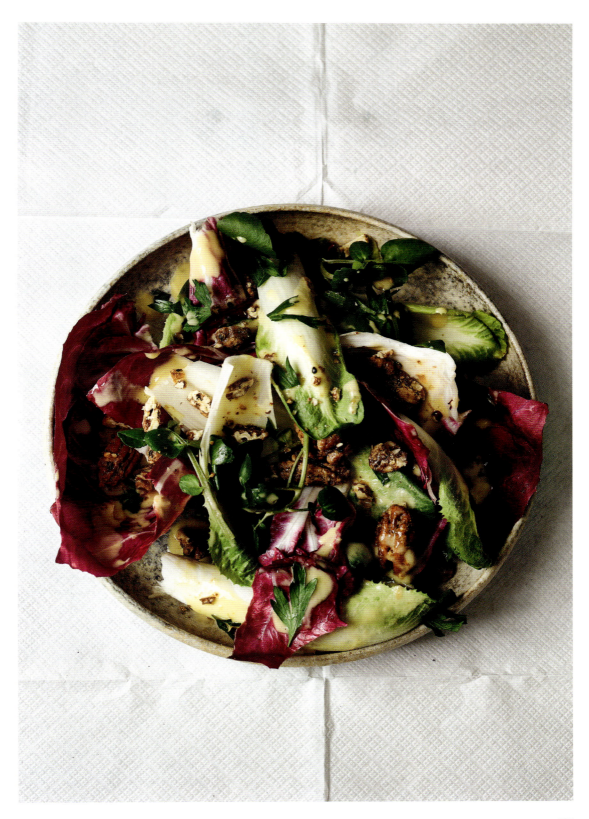

MAINS

Butternut Squash, Broccolini & Lentils with Charred Leek & Miso-Tahini Yogurt

One of the few recipes I've committed to memory is an Ottolenghi roasted butternut squash and red onion situation. I've made it so many times that it's now instinctual and driven by taste. And as my taste has evolved, so has my version, which you will find below.

Here, butternut squash and broccolini are roasted with miso and maple syrup, served with lemony lentils on a bed of miso-tahini yogurt, and sprinkled with charred leeks, fresh parsley, and quick-pickled red onions and chiles. It's a side dish that has forced its way into the mains category and a perfect meal-prep dish, as leftovers make a great midday salad. I often mix the roasted veg together to be eaten in a sandwich.

All elements of the salad can be made ahead of time, but it's best to assemble just before eating. I don't want to say every meal requires carbs, but I'd eat this with some crusty bread, Sauercaccia (see page 156) or Kimchi & Cheddar Biscuits (see page 180).

PREP TIME: 25 MINUTES | COOK TIME: 35–40 MINUTES

Preheat the oven to 350°F (180°C) and set up two oven shelves. The leeks and the other vegetables will bake at the same time but on separate baking sheets. Line two baking sheets with parchment paper.

Put the leeks on one lined baking sheet and toss with 2 teaspoons of the olive oil, the smoked paprika, and a pinch of salt. This goes on the top shelf in your oven.

Put the butternut squash and broccoli on the second lined baking sheet. Combine the remaining olive oil with the red miso and maple syrup in a small bowl, pour over the vegetables, and mix well: Using your hands helps to ensure the vegetables are evenly coated. Arrange them in a single layer.

Ingredients and recipe continue on the next page

Serves 4–6

- 1 leek, trimmed, washed, and cut into 5-cm (2-in) segments
- 3 tbsp, plus 2 tsp olive oil
- ½ tsp smoked paprika
- salt and pepper
- 400g (14oz) butternut squash, peeled and cut in half, then into 5-mm (¼-in) slices
- 200g (7oz) broccolini, cut into 5-cm (2-in) segments
- 2 tbsp red miso
- 1 tbsp maple syrup or clear honey
- 200g (1 cup) cooked brown lentils

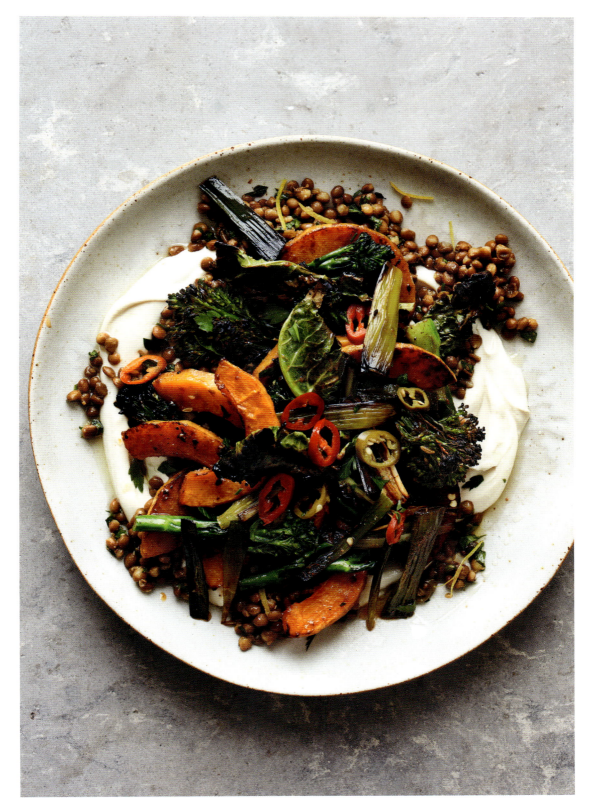

Bake both sheets of vegetables for 35–40 minutes until the leeks are golden brown and crunchy (but not burnt), the butternut squash fork tender, and the broccolini has a slight char.

While the vegetables are in the oven, combine the lentils, lemon zest and juice, and chopped parsley and season with salt and pepper.

To make the miso-tahini yogurt, whisk all of the ingredients together in a bowl until smooth.

Assemble the dish on a large plate: Spread over the miso-tahini yogurt, followed by the lentils, roasted butternut and broccolini, and the roasted leeks on top. Garnish with a generous sprinkle of pickled red onions and/or chiles, chopped parsley, and finish with a drizzle of extra virgin olive oil.

zest of 1 lemon and 2 tbsp lemon juice

handful of fresh parsley (about 10g/0.33oz), roughly chopped

FOR THE MISO-TAHINI YOGURT

125g (½ cup) full-fat yogurt

65g (¼ cup) tahini

2 tbsp Kombucha Citrus Syrup (see page 138), maple syrup or clear honey

3 tbsp lemon juice

2 tsp white miso

TO SERVE

Quick-Pickled Red Onions (see page 114) and/or Quick-Pickled Kombucha Chiles (see page 112)

5 sprigs of fresh parsley, roughly chopped

extra virgin olive oil

Chickpea & Sauerkraut Salad

This weeknight salad is the definition of a kitchen-pantry rustle up. Any flavor of sauerkraut will work here, so if you're like me and have a variety of spice combinations fermenting away in your kitchen, the possibilities are endless. Using sauerkraut as an ingredient offers not only a zing of flavor, but also adds texture (and is a great way to use up ferments to make way for more projects). Canned chickpeas are what we normally have in our pantry, but feel free to use any of your favorite canned beans, such as lima, black, or kidney beans.

Taking this as your starting point, you can bulk it up with roasted vegetables, add Miso Parm Croutons (see page 194), Curried Crispy Lima Beans (see page 198) or, as I often do, serve it on a bed of arugula.

PREP TIME: 10 MINUTES

Serves 4

700g (4¼ cups) canned chickpeas, drained

200g (1⅓ cups) sauerkraut, including residual brine

60g (2½ cups) fresh leafy herbs, such as cilantro, parsley, or dill, chopped

zest and juice of 1 lemon

salt and pepper

100g (¼ cup plus 3 tbsp) feta, crumbled into bite-size pieces

In your serving bowl, combine the chickpeas, sauerkraut, and chopped herbs. Give this a good mix.
 Dress with the lemon zest and juice and season with salt and pepper.
 Sprinkle the feta on top.
 This salad keeps well in the fridge for up to 2 days.

MAINS

Miso Pesto Pasta Salad with Chili Crisp Balsamic Roasted Tomatoes

This quick weeknight meal is a feast of layered umami: not only from the miso in the pesto but also from the tomatoes, slow roasted in a sticky, sweet dressing of balsamic and chili crisp. Both elements can be made independently—the pesto is a super-quick vegan version—but the addition of the tomatoes elevates this dish. It's also great at room temperature, so a perfect meal for picnics or to prepare for weekday work lunches. For additional freshness, throw in arugula, watercress, or chopped kale (massaged with a bit of salt and extra virgin olive oil), or a few handfuls of sauerkraut, brine squeezed out.

PREP TIME: 15 MINUTES | COOK TIME: 15 MINUTES

To make the pesto, put all of the ingredients into a food processor and blitz to your desired consistency. I prefer a rough-textured pesto that is not too puréed. Adjust the seasoning with salt—but additional seasoning will come from the tomatoes.

To make the chili crisp balsamic roasted tomatoes, preheat the oven to 450°F (230°C) and line a baking sheet with parchment paper. Put all of the ingredients for the tomatoes on the lined baking sheet and roast for 15 minutes. Give the tray an occasional shake, and after 7–8 minutes, use a wooden spoon to smash some of the tomatoes—the beginning of a jammy sauce. Once the tomatoes are done, use a metal spatula to scrape off all of the residual bits from the paper and mix them back into the sauce.

While the tomatoes are roasting, toast the cashews in a dry pan over a low heat until lightly browned, around 3 minutes. Roughly crush the cashews—rugged is best. If you do not have a mortar and pestle, crush them on a cutting board, using the bottom of a pan.

Cook the pasta in a pot of boiling salted water according to the package instructions. Drain, reserving 120ml (½ cup) of the pasta cooking water.

Return the drained pasta to the pot, add the pesto, and mix until fully combined. You may need to add some of the reserved pasta cooking water to loosen it. Serve with a dollop of the roasted tomatoes on top of the pasta, followed by the crushed cashews, sliced basil, and a lemon wedge.

Serves 4

1 tbsp unsalted cashews
300–350g (10.5–12oz) pasta (my favorites are casarecce, penne, or fusilli)
handful of fresh basil leaves, thinly sliced, to garnish
lemon wedges to serve

FOR THE PESTO

40g (⅓ cup) unsalted cashews
70g (3 cups) basil
1 large garlic clove, peeled
1 tbsp red miso
60ml (¼ cup) extra virgin olive oil

FOR THE CHILI CRISP BALSAMIC ROASTED TOMATOES

500g (1lb 2oz) cherry tomatoes
1 tbsp olive oil
2 tbsp chili crisp or chili oil (Laoganma is my favorite brand)
2 tbsp white sesame seeds
1 tbsp balsamic vinegar

SPECIAL EQUIPMENT: food processor

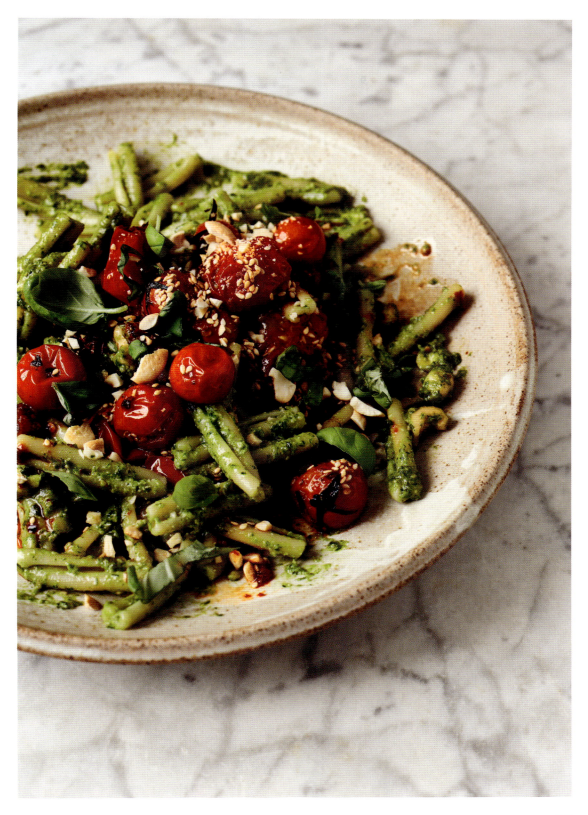

Fennel & Arugula Miso Caesar with Charred Miso Parm Croutons

Maybe it's just me but I find there's something glamorous about making a Caesar salad. I remember being blown away by the layering of umami when my husband made me a Caesar when we first moved to London. Growing up, I always found Caesar salads a bit gloopy, the rich dressing (often premade from grocery stores) laid thick on romaine. I'm pleased to know making a much better version at home is as easy as blitzing a few ingredients together.

This vegetarian version of a Caesar dressing swaps out anchovies for miso, and I like pairing it against the texture of fennel and bitterness of arugula. However, you can go classic with romaine or gem lettuce. The croutons serve a few purposes: even more texture to enjoy, umami amplification, and extra bitterness to offset the richness of the dressing.

This recipe makes approximately 240ml (1 cup) of dressing, which is intentionally thick. It's more than you'll need for one salad but you'll thank me later, as this aioli-like dressing keeps for up to a week in the fridge. Use it for more salads, or as a spread on a sandwich, which is particularly delicious.

PREP TIME: 20 MINUTES | COOK TIME: 10 MINUTES

Put all of the ingredients for the dressing (except the olive oil) into a food processor and blitz. Slowly add the olive oil and continue to blitz until emulsified. Keep the dressing in the fridge until needed.

To make the croutons, preheat the oven to 375°F (190°C). In a bowl, mix together the olive oil, red miso, and Parmesan. Slice the bread into crouton-size pieces and add them to the mixture, tossing to combine.

Arrange the croutons on a baking sheet in a single layer and bake for 10 minutes, or until they are nicely browned with some charred bits. The sugar in the miso will burn, so keep an eye out for this if your oven runs hot.

To assemble the salad, put the arugula and fennel in a large mixing bowl, add 1–2 tablespoons of the dressing, and toss well. If you find the dressing too thick, thin it out with ½ teaspoon of apple cider vinegar. Always start with a small amount of the dressing: You can add more once the salad is mixed.

Plate the salad and garnish with the croutons and shavings of Parmesan, season with freshly cracked black pepper, and serve.

Serves 2

150g (5oz) arugula
1 fennel bulb, thinly sliced
Parmesan shavings to garnish

FOR THE MISO CAESAR DRESSING

2 egg yolks
1 garlic clove, peeled and grated
2 tsp red miso
1 tsp Dijon mustard
1 tsp apple cider vinegar
200ml (¾ cup plus 1 tbsp) extra virgin olive oil

FOR THE MISO PARM CROUTONS

2 tbsp olive oil
1 tbsp red miso
1 tbsp grated Parmesan
100g (3.5oz) crusty sourdough

SPECIAL EQUIPMENT: food processor

Kimchi Caponata

With every trip to Japan, I'm always blown away by the creativity and innovation in izakaya (small plates) cuisine. On my last visit, I got in the habit of ordering almost anything that included kimchi, which probably isn't surprising. What may surprise you, however, is how kimchi intensifies in umami and sweetness as you cook it. Some of my favorite ways to eat kimchi are in cooked form: kimchi pancakes, kimchi fried rice, kimchi jjigae. Now enter my fun fusion contribution to this list: kimchi caponata. It can be eaten as a standalone dish, alongside your favorite pasta or with crusty bread, or as an excellent side dish. Like traditional caponata, this is something you can make in advance and let cool to room temperature before consuming, so you can focus on the rest of the meal.

PREP TIME: 25 MINUTES | COOK TIME: 35–40 MINUTES

Preheat the oven to 425°F (220°C).

Chop the eggplants and zucchinis into 2-cm (¾-inch) cubes and put them in a bowl (the small size will allow them to cook quickly and become crisp). Stir the salt into the vegetables and set aside for 15 minutes, occasionally giving them a mix.

Remove excess liquid from the eggplant and zucchini by giving them a gentle squeeze, then put them back into the bowl. Add the olive oil and stir, ensuring everything is coated. Season with salt and pepper. Put the vegetables in a single layer on a large baking sheet and bake for 35–40 minutes. Give them a shake every now and then to ensure they cook evenly. The vegetables will shrink considerably.

While they are in the oven, heat a saucepan over a medium heat with a drizzle of olive oil and fry the kimchi, onion, tomatoes, garlic, and capers for 5–7 minutes, until the onion has softened and the tomatoes are cooked down. Add the sugar and vinegar, turn off the heat, and mix to combine, dissolving the sugar in the residual heat. Cover and set aside until the eggplant and zucchini are done.

Once the eggplants and zucchinis are nicely browned and out of the oven, add them to the saucepan. Stir well and serve, or even better, wait until the next day to allow the flavors to really meld.

Serves 2–4

2 eggplants, about 600g (1lb 5oz) total weight

2 zucchinis, about 400g (14oz) total weight

1 tsp salt, plus extra for seasoning

100ml (¼ cup plus 3 tbsp) olive oil, plus extra for drizzling

black pepper

150g (1 cup) kimchi, roughly chopped

1 onion, peeled and thinly sliced

225g (8oz) tomatoes, chopped

3 garlic cloves, peeled and finely chopped

3 tbsp capers, drained

1 tsp sugar

2 tbsp red wine vinegar

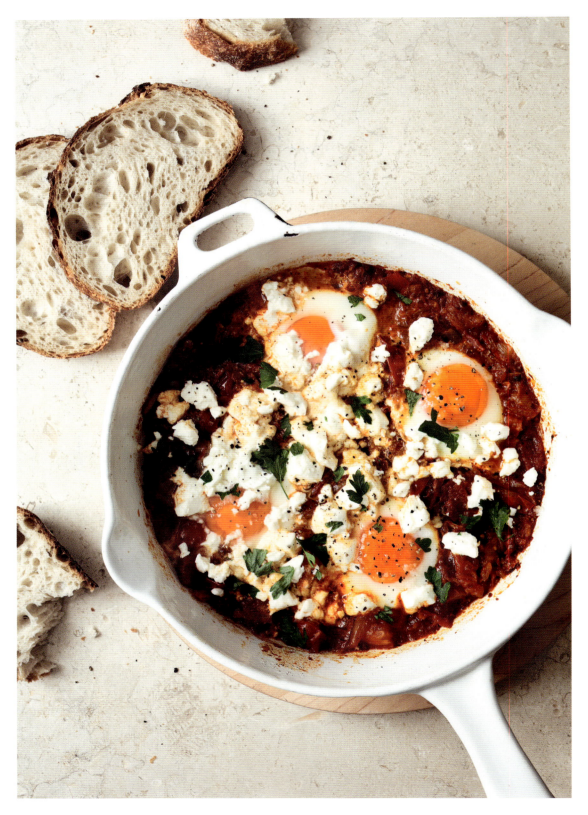

Kimchi & Harissa Shakshuka

This is no traditional shakshuka. For how quick and easy this meal is (under 30 minutes), it packs a punch. Not only in the layers of spice and heat coming from the kimchi and the harissa paste, but also in the way this combination works against the simple canvas of an egg: a perfect foil to the salty tang of the feta, which intensifies as it cooks. The amount of feta you use is totally up to you, but I do love that tart hit of feta and creaminess with my morning eggs.

Enjoy all of these flavors and textures with crusty bread. Cold leftovers are incredible as an open sandwich with Miso Hummus (see page 172) and some Pineapple & Scotch Bonnet Hot Sauce (see page 48).

PREP TIME: 10 MINUTES | COOK TIME: 20 MINUTES

Heat the olive oil in a medium frying pan (for which you have a lid) over a medium heat, then add the tomatoes and kimchi and cook, uncovered, for 5–7 minutes.

Add the harissa, fish sauce, and sugar and 200ml (¾ cup plus 1 tablespoon) of water and simmer gently, uncovered, for 5–10 minutes, until the sauce has thickened.

Crack 4 eggs into the tomato kimchi mixture and crumble the feta on top.

Put the lid on and cook for a further 5 minutes or until the eggs are cooked to your liking. Garnish with chopped parsley, season with freshly cracked black pepper, and dive in with some crusty bread.

Serves 2

1 tbsp olive oil

250g (9oz) vine tomatoes, chopped

150g (1 cup) kimchi, drained and chopped

1 tbsp harissa

1 tsp fish sauce

1 tsp sugar

4 medium eggs

100g (¼ cup plus 3 tbsp) feta, crumbled

handful of fresh parsley, chopped, to garnish

Green Mean Bean Miso Soup with Curried Crispy Lima Beans

Whenever I'm feeling the need for some healthy nourishment, I make this soup. The soup on its own uses pantry staples and can be done in 15–20 minutes. The curried crispy lima beans take more time to bake, and can be excluded if you're in a rush, but they really add a nice texture and warmth to the dish. And it's all quite pretty: As the kale is just barely cooked, the soup retains a bright green color while the lima beans add that perfect creaminess. Both the soup and crispy lima beans are delicious on their own, but even better together!

PREP TIME: 15 MINUTES | COOK TIME: 20–45 MINUTES

First make the curried crispy lima beans. Preheat the oven to 425°F (220°C). Use a clean kitchen towel or paper towel to absorb moisture from the beans; you want them to be as dry as possible. Toss the dried beans with the oil, curry powder, turmeric, cayenne, and salt and then spread them on a baking sheet. Bake for 20–45 minutes until golden brown and crispy. The exact time will depend on the beans you use and your oven, so start checking after 20 minutes.

To make the soup, heat the olive oil in a heavy-bottomed pan over a medium-high heat. Add the shallot and fry for 2–3 minutes until softened. Add the garlic and cook for a further 1–2 minutes.

Add the kale and stir until the color changes to a vibrant green as it softens. Add the stock and the lima beans, including the liquid from the can, and bring to a gentle simmer until the kale is cooked (it should be done within a few minutes).

Pour the soup into a blender and blitz until smooth. I like this soup to be quite thick, but if you prefer a thinner soup, add more stock.

Pour the soup back into the pan and stir in the miso, allowing the residual heat to dissolve it. Taste and adjust the seasoning: You can add more miso but be sure to fully dissolve it. Serve the soup drizzled with olive oil and seasoned with freshly cracked black pepper, with the crispy lima beans in a separate bowl to be added at the table.

This freezes well if you have leftovers.

Serves 4–6

- 1 tbsp olive oil
- 1 shallot, diced
- 3 garlic cloves, peeled and finely chopped
- 200g (7oz) curly kale (or similar leafy greens such as lacinato kale or spinach), chopped
- 500ml (2 cups plus 1 tbsp) chicken or vegetable stock
- 375g (2¼ cups) canned lima beans (or similar creamy beans such as white beans or chickpeas)
- 2 tbsp red miso
- extra virgin olive oil to serve

FOR THE CURRIED CRISPY LIMA BEANS

- 125g (¾ cup) canned lima beans, drained
- 1 tbsp olive oil
- 2 tsp curry powder
- ½ tsp ground turmeric
- 1 tsp cayenne
- ½ tsp salt

SPECIAL EQUIPMENT: blender

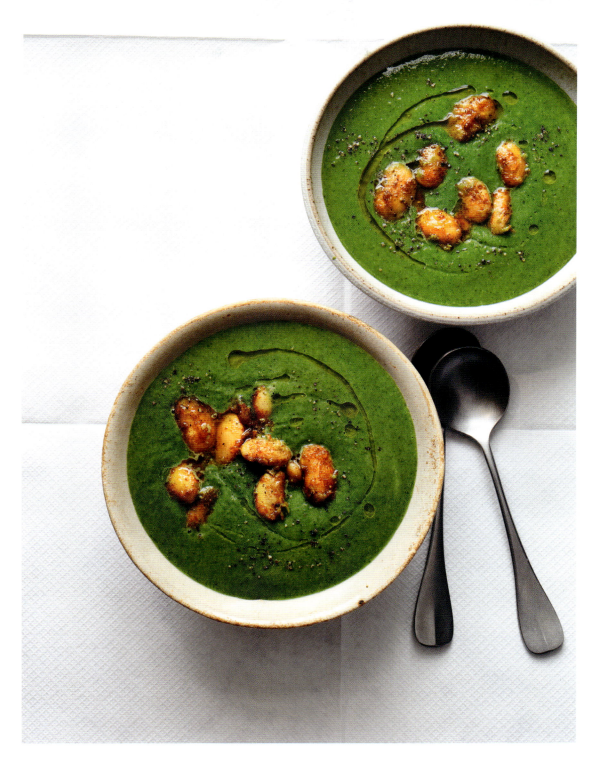

Kimchi & Feta Spanakopita with Gochujang Butter

Next time you need something to bring to a friends' gathering or picnic, make this dish. It plays on traditional spanakopita but is intense with kimchi umami. Spanakopita has always been one of my favorite snacks and was my top choice of baked goods when my mom would ask for weekend requests.

I've made a few variations on a ferment-forward spanakopita using different lactofermented greens, but this kimchi version is my definite winner. There are a lot of strong flavors here, but it works. The kimchi really shines, its flavor intensified and balanced against the sharp and creamy feta. The combination of sesame oil and spinach reminds me of a Korean spinach namul, but then that phyllo shatters, crisp and brown with a gochujang butter.

I used a 23 x 33-cm (9 x 13-in) oven-safe dish. You can use a different size but may need to adjust the timing slightly. Generally, keep an eye on the spanakopita when baking—each oven is different. It's also a great recipe to make ahead.

PREP TIME: 30 MINUTES | COOK TIME: 45–60 MINUTES

Wash the spinach and put it into a pan with its residual water; cook over a medium-low heat just until it begins to wilt. Tip it into a colander and leave to cool slightly, then squeeze it to remove excess water. If using fresh spinach, you should end up with about 180–200g (6–7oz) once squeezed. You can use frozen spinach, but ensure you end up with 180–200g (6–7oz) once squeezed to remove excess water.

Heat the olive oil in a pan over a medium heat. Add the onions and a pinch of salt and cook for 3–5 minutes until jammy and slightly browned. Add the chopped kimchi and cook for a further 5 minutes. The residual kimchi brine should deglaze the pan but keep an eye on it in case it starts to stick. Once the kimchi begins to caramelize, remove from the heat.

In a mixing bowl, combine the onion and kimchi mixture with the squeezed spinach. Crumble in the feta, then add the sesame oil and a few grinds of black pepper.

Serves 8

500g (1lb 2oz) fresh spinach

1 tbsp olive oil

2 onions, peeled and finely diced

salt and pepper

250g (1⅔ cups) kimchi, roughly chopped

200g (¾ cup) feta, crumbled

2 tsp toasted sesame oil

75g (⅓ cup) unsalted butter

1 tbsp gochujang

1 pack of phyllo pastry (7 sheets of phyllo), fully defrosted

1 egg, beaten

black sesame seeds

SPECIAL EQUIPMENT: 23 x 33-cm (9 x 13-in) oven-safe dish

Preheat the oven to 375°F (190°C).

Melt the butter and gochujang in a small saucepan over a low heat and whisk until fully combined. Brush the base and sides of your oven-safe dish with the gochujang butter.

When using phyllo pastry, work quickly as it can be fragile and dries out easily. Layer two sheets of phyllo pastry in the dish, letting the pastry overhang the sides, and brush with a generous amount of the gochujang butter. Add another two layers of phyllo, brushing the top layer with more gochujang butter.

Spread the kimchi spinach mixture over the phyllo pastry in a thick layer.

Cover with two more phyllo sheets, brush with gochujang butter, then lay the final sheet of phyllo on top and brush with more gochujang butter.

Fold in and crinkle the sides, and brush it all with the remaining gochujang butter. Brush the beaten egg over the pastry, which will give it a nice shine. Sprinkle on some black sesame seeds.

Bake the spanakopita for 45–60 minutes until golden brown. Let it cool for 15–20 minutes before cutting and eating.

Once cooled, this can be frozen.

Plant-Based Zero-Waste Green Curry

This is THE definition of a fridge-raid meal, the star of the show being the homemade Zero-Waste Green Paste (see page 40). Use any combination of vegetables, which is important for a good everyday curry. It's versatile, easy, and a good way to clear out some fridge real estate.

I'd aim to use mixed vegetables that offer variety in texture and color. In the photo, I've gone with a combination of sweet potato, eggplant, broccoli florets, and fresh shiitake. Other options include baby potatoes, green beans, carrots, cherry tomatoes, baby corn, and red or yellow pepper.

This takes inspiration from Thai green curry in both flavor and process but has been considerably simplified. The amount of green paste can be adjusted (more will yield a darker and spicier curry). I like how veg-forward this dish is, but you can add tofu (warmed in the curry) or chicken thigh (cut into bite-size pieces and cooked at a simmer in the curry for the last 10 minutes of cooking) for protein.

PREP TIME: 15 MINUTES | COOK TIME: 25 MINUTES

In a heavy-bottomed saucepan, heat the oil over a low heat. Add the paste and let it cook off for 3 minutes, stirring to ensure it doesn't stick and burn.

Deglaze by pouring in all of the coconut milk and 240ml (1 cup) of water and stirring well. Add the lemongrass and lime leaves and bring to a simmer.

Add any vegetables that need a longer cooking time (such as potato or sweet potato) and simmer over a low heat for 5–7 minutes, then add the remaining vegetables.

Add the miso, sugar, and soy sauce and leave to simmer for 5–7 minutes.

Remove the lemongrass and lime leaves if you prefer—I don't mind biting into a lime leaf, but it can be unpleasant to encounter an unruly smashed lemongrass stalk.

Serve with rice and garnish with fresh herbs, thinly sliced chile, and the mandatory good squeeze of lime juice.

Serves 4–6

2 tbsp vegetable oil

150–250g (5–9oz) Zero-Waste Green Paste (see page 40)

two 400-ml (14-oz) cans full-fat coconut milk

2 lemongrass stalks, bruised and bashed with the back of a knife

8 makrut lime leaves, bruised

approximately 550g (1lb 3oz) colorful vegetables (see above), cut into small bite-size pieces

1 tbsp red miso

1 tbsp plus 1½ tsp sugar

1 tbsp light soy sauce

rice to serve

TO SERVE

fresh herbs

fresh chile, thinly sliced, or Quick-Pickled Kombucha Chiles (see page 112)

lime wedges

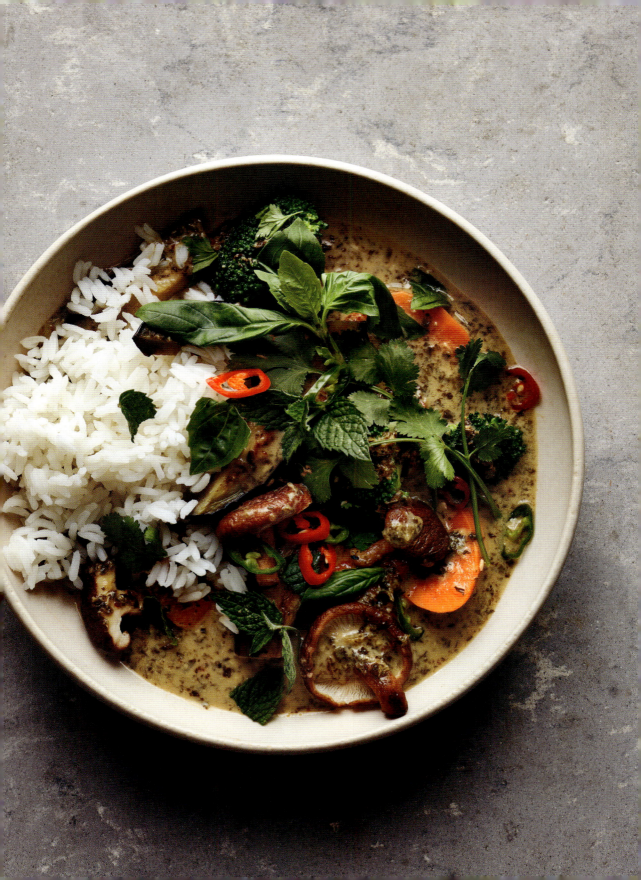

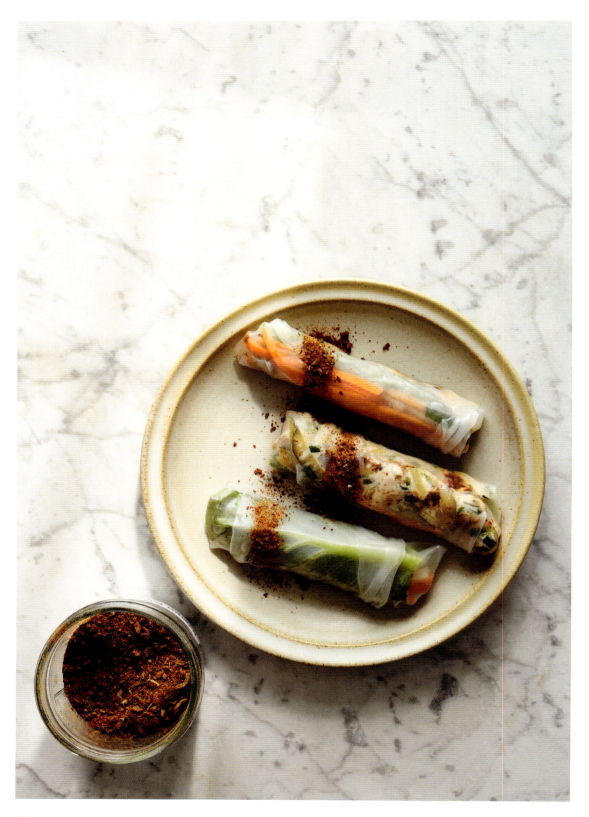

Sweet Pickle Tuna Summer Rolls

When I'm craving a light but satisfying meal, I gravitate toward summer rolls. Using rice paper may seem intimidating and requires a bit of practice, but even if they don't come out perfectly, they will still be delicious! You can have fun with the filling—they're a great way to consume a variety of vegetables and pickles—but don't try to pack in too many if you're new to this technique. The Zucchini Bread & Butter Pickles are the main source of flavor. However, you could also add extra pickles—a favorite of mine is the Kombucha-Pickled Carrot & Daikon (see page 117). The kimchi sprinkles are a fun addition to the rolls, adding both a spicy umami punch and a bit of crunch, reminiscent of crispy fried shallots. I've also included an optional simple Nước chấm recipe if you fancy!

PREP TIME: 15–20 MINUTES

Put the tuna into a mixing bowl with the mayo, pickles, and green onions. Season with salt and pepper and set aside.

Working quickly, dunk one sheet of rice paper into a bowl of water for 15–20 seconds. The rice paper won't seem pliable but trust the process.

Place the rice paper onto a clean kitchen towel. Put one gem lettuce leaf on the bottom third of the rice paper closest to you, with the rib side of the leaf facing down—this provides structure. Trim the lettuce so there's space on both sides for easy rolling.

Spoon about an eighth of the tuna salad mixture onto the lettuce, followed by 1 tablespoon of the kimchi sprinkles. You could add more vegetables or pickles/ferments, but don't add too much otherwise it might fall apart.

Fold the rice paper edge closest to you up and over the filling. Gently roll it over to ensure the filling is enclosed, then fold in the sides and finish rolling it up. Try to keep the filling as compact as possible. Repeat with the remaining rice paper sheets and filling.

To serve, cut the rolls in half and enjoy! I like dunking them into more kimchi sprinkles with each bite. If you'd also like to serve them with a dipping sauce, simply mix together all of the sauce ingredients with 120ml (½ cup) water and enjoy!

Makes 8 summer rolls

two 145-g (5-oz) cans of tuna (in brine or oil), drained

2 tbsp mayonnaise

125g (4.5oz) Zucchini Bread & Butter Pickles (see page 109), roughly chopped

3 green onions, trimmed and thinly sliced

salt and pepper

8 sheets rice paper

8 gem lettuce leaves

8 tbsp Kimchi Sprinkles (see page 76)

FOR THE NƯỚC CHẤM DIPPING SAUCE (OPTIONAL)

50g (¼ cup) sugar or honey

60ml (¼ cup) lime juice or Kombucha Citrus Syrup (see page 138)—if you use the syrup, decrease the sugar content

60ml (¼ cup) fish sauce

1 tbsp Quick-Pickled Kombucha Chiles (see page 112)

Miso Fishermen's Pie

I discovered fish pie only when I moved to London. It reminds me of two things: Japanese cream stew, and clam chowder from Legal Sea Foods, a well-known restaurant chain in Boston, Massachusetts. As newlyweds, my parents went on dates there and always spoke fondly of that clam chowder. When I went to college nearby, I loved it too, but then life took me further afield. This dish triggers those stories, a comforting feeling of home in a single bite.

And why is this called a fishermen's pie? Blame my family: They struggled with the concept of a fish pie. So let's call this a happy medium from across the pond. This is easy to make ahead of time and reheat on the day of serving.

PREP TIME: 25 MINUTES | COOK TIME: 45 MINUTES

Bring a pot of water to a boil and simmer the potatoes for 15–20 minutes until fork tender. Drain, then mash the potatoes with the butter and cheese, and set aside.

Warm the milk and sliced ginger in a saucepan and bring to a gentle simmer. Add the seafood and cook over a medium-low heat for around 3 minutes or until the fish is cooked through and opaque. Remove the poached fish and reserve the poaching liquid. Preheat the oven to 425°F (220°C).

To make the béchamel, melt the butter in a medium saucepan over a medium heat and stir-fry the green onions until they turn deep green. Add the flour and cook for 2 minutes, stirring vigorously. Gradually add the reserved poaching liquid and cook for 5–10 minutes, stirring continuously to ensure there are no clumps of flour, until the liquid has thickened.

Take the béchamel off the heat, gently stir in the miso until it dissolves, then add the poached fish.

Spoon the fish mixture into the baking dish. Add the mashed potatoes and use an offset spatula to spread the potatoes completely and evenly over the fish.

Bake the pie in the oven for 20–25 minutes until the potato topping is browned and crisp. Serve immediately. Once cooled, this freezes well.

Serves 4–6

1kg (2.25lbs) potatoes, peeled and quartered

50g (4 tbsp) unsalted butter

200g (1¾ cups) cheddar, grated

400ml (1⅔ cups) whole milk

50g (1.75oz) fresh ginger, peeled and thinly sliced

450g (1lb) mixed seafood (any combination of salmon, smoked haddock, and cod or hake, or really any seafood combination you like, including some shellfish), cut into large bite-size chunks

FOR THE BÉCHAMEL

30g (2 tbsp) unsalted butter

4 green onions, trimmed and thinly sliced

30g (¼ cup) all-purpose flour

3 tbsp red miso

SPECIAL EQUIPMENT: 23 x 33-cm (9 x 13-in) baking dish

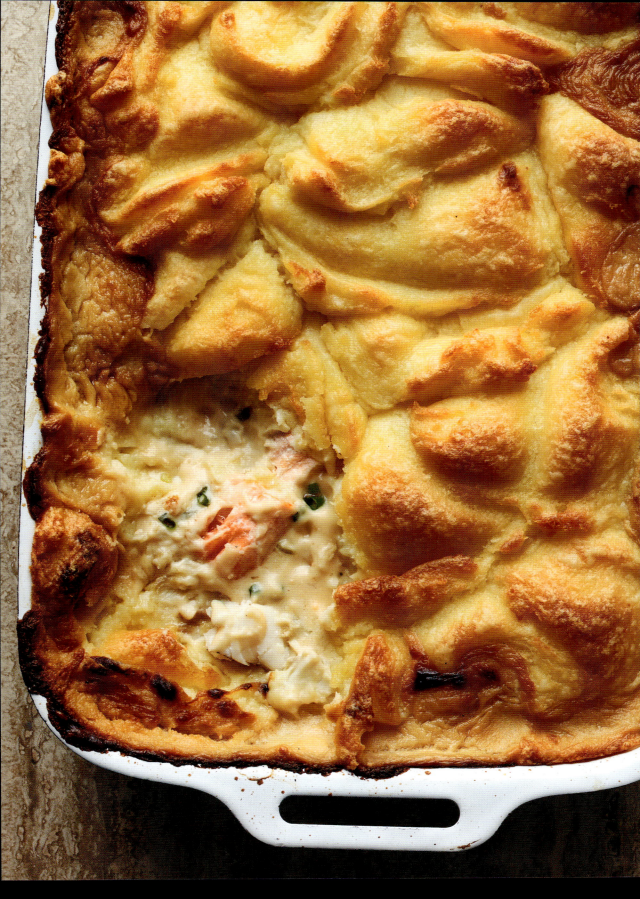

Fried Fish Sandwich with Pickles & Miso Aioli

This is my Platonic ideal of a sandwich: freshly fried, golden panko-coated fish fillets on a toasted brioche bun with a thick miso aioli and pickled carrot and daikon. And some gem lettuce, of course.

You can add more pickles (kimchi would be delicious), more sauces—Everyday Hot Sauce (see page 45) or even tonkatsu sauce—but don't say I didn't warn you how messy it can be!

Feel free to scale this up, especially if you want to take advantage of deep-frying—leftover fried fish is good both at room temperature and reheated in the oven.

PREP TIME: 10 MINUTES | COOK TIME: 15 MINUTES

Cut the fish fillets in half, so you have four pieces of fish. Pat the fish dry with paper towels and season generously with salt and pepper.

Fill a deep cast-iron pan or wok with vegetable oil (no more than one-third full for safety) and turn the heat to high. If using a deep-fat fryer, heat the oil to 350°F (180°C).

While the oil is heating, prepare the frying stations: Put the flour in a shallow bowl; put the panko in a separate shallow bowl; whisk the eggs in another bowl. Line a dish with paper towels.

One at a time, dredge a fillet first in flour, then in egg, and finally in the panko. Really pack on the panko. Put the breaded fish on a plate while you repeat the process with the remaining fillets.

To check that the oil is hot enough, drop a small amount of the panko into the oil: If it immediately starts to float and sizzle, it's ready to start frying. Do not overcrowd the pan. Cook the fillets for no more than 3 minutes on each side, until both sides are golden brown. Drain on the lined dish to absorb excess oil and immediately season with salt.

To assemble, smear a healthy dollop of miso dressing on the bottom bun, followed by the gem lettuce. Then the fried fish, with a generous helping of pickled carrot and daikon on top. If you like, melt some American cheese on top, then add more miso dressing on the top bun and dive in.

Makes 4 sandwiches

2 white fish fillets, such as haddock or cod, about 250g (9oz) total weight

salt and pepper

vegetable oil for deep-frying

70g (½ cup plus 1 tbsp) all-purpose flour

70g (⅔ cup) panko bread crumbs

2 eggs, beaten

4 brioche buns, toasted

Miso Caesar Dressing (see page 194)

gem lettuce (one leaf per sandwich)

Kombucha-Pickled Carrot & Daikon (see page 117)

American cheese (optional: if feeling naughty, one slice per sandwich)

SPECIAL EQUIPMENT: deep-fat fryer (optional)

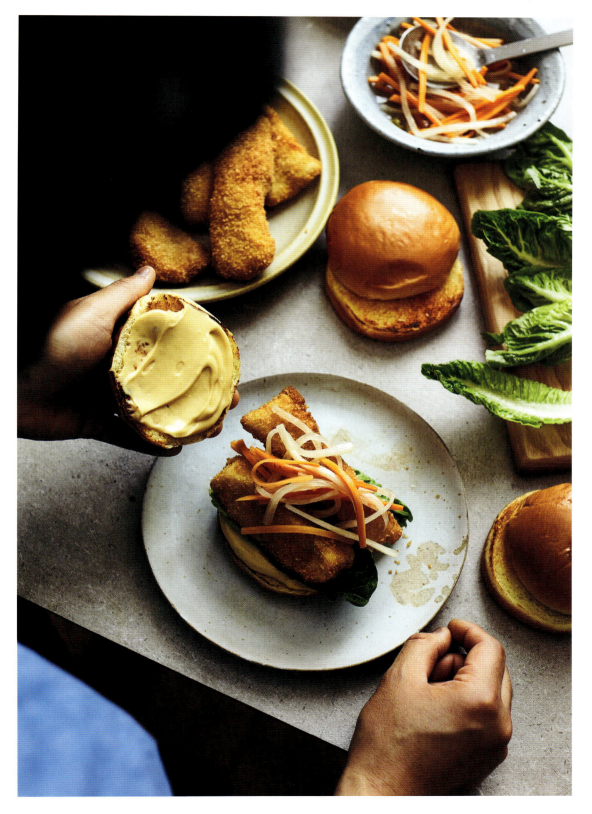

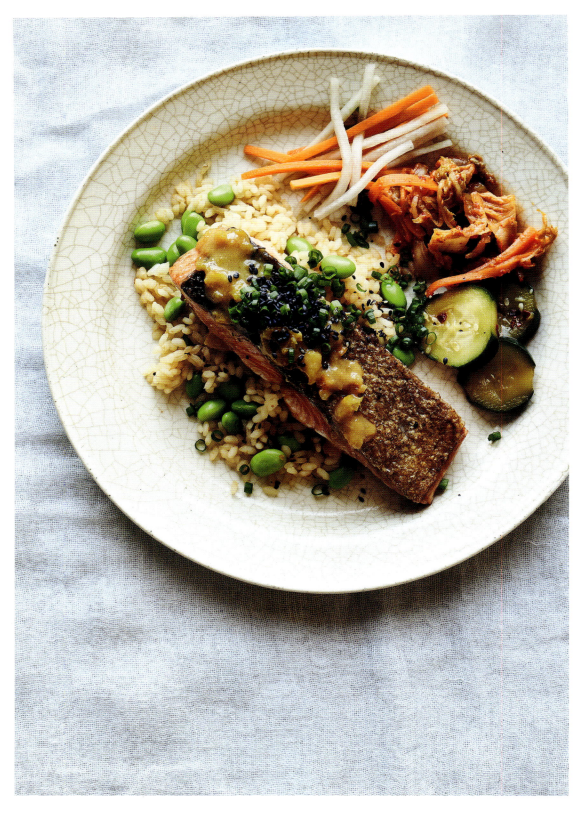

Citrus-Miso Salmon & Edamame Rice

This is a quick meal, pretty much limited to the time it takes to cook rice. The star of the dish is the crispy skinned salmon, which is more than doable if you follow the process below. The beauty of this dish is in the combination of the various elements: freshly cooked rice lightly seasoned with miso and studded with edamame, a thick citrusy miso sauce on top of the crispy salmon skin, and a variety of pickles. Using the preserved citrus from the Kombucha Citrus Syrup (see page 138) adds a marmalade-like bite and is a great way to use up a by-product of that ferment.

When I made this for my parents, they recounted how this was really their ideal meal: simple in process, a variety of textures and flavors, especially when you add whatever pickles you have fermenting or pickling, and packed with umami thanks to the layering of miso throughout the dish.

PREP TIME: 20 MINUTES | COOK TIME: 15 MINUTES

Lightly salt both sides of the salmon fillets and set aside for 15 minutes.

While the fish is salting, start cooking the rice—use your preferred method, and add the frozen edamame and red miso.

Use a paper towel to absorb excess water from the salted salmon fillets. Put the fillets skin side down on a cold nonstick frying pan; cook over a medium heat for 5 minutes, using a fish spatula to press down on the flesh, then leave the fish undisturbed for 10 minutes. After that time the flesh should be fairly cooked through and the skin should release from the pan. Turn off the heat and flip, allowing the residual heat to cook the other side of the fish.

To make the sauce, whisk together the preserved citrus, kombucha citrus syrup, white miso, rice vinegar, and sesame oil. Season with salt and pepper.

Assemble your plate of food: Pile on some rice, add the salmon fillet, skin side up, spoon on the citrus miso sauce, and garnish with green onions and sesame seeds. Serve with a variety of pickles.

Serves 2

2 skin-on salmon fillets
salt
70–100g (⅓–½ cup) short-grain rice (white or brown)
100g (¾ cup plus 2 tbsp) frozen edamame
1 tbsp red miso
2 green onions, trimmed and thinly sliced, to garnish
black sesame seeds to serve
pickles to serve

FOR THE CITRUS MISO SAUCE

1 slice of preserved citrus from Kombucha Citrus Syrup (see page 138), finely chopped
1 tbsp Kombucha Citrus Syrup
1 tbsp white miso
1 tbsp rice vinegar
1 tsp toasted sesame oil
salt and pepper

Ten-Minute Miso Peanut Butter Kimchi Noodles

Be it after a long work day or the morning after a big night out, I crave carbs, preferably flavorful and very quick to make. This is my go-to dish in these and many other situations. The sauce is made entirely from pantry staples, with nutty creaminess coming from the peanut butter and complexity in umami and spice from the miso and kimchi—both the brine and pickles.

I often hear of people not knowing what to do with their leftover kimchi brine. Remember that it can be treated as a separate ingredient; here, it both loosens the sauce and adds a lot of flavor and tang. If you have other fermented brines on hand—from sauerkraut, or wet brines from hot sauces—use them, and adjust to your own personal taste.

PREP TIME: 5 MINUTES | COOK TIME: 5–10 MINUTES

Prepare your noodles or pasta according to the package instructions.

For the last 3 minutes of the noodle cooking time, add the asparagus. A minute later, add the bok choy.

In a large mixing bowl, whisk together all of the sauce ingredients.

When the noodles and vegetables are ready, drain and add them to the mixing bowl, reserving some of the noodle cooking water in case you need to loosen the sauce.

Garnish with green onion and sesame seeds.

Serves 1

80–100g (3–3.5oz) dried noodles (instant noodles or spaghetti are my favorites for this)

FOR THE SAUCE

1 tbsp peanut butter (chunky or smooth)

1 tbsp red miso

1½ tsp clear honey or maple syrup

1 tsp coarse gochugaru

1 tsp toasted sesame oil

3 tbsp kimchi brine

2 tbsp kimchi, thinly sliced

TO SERVE

asparagus, cut into thirds

bok choy, leaves separated

cucumber, julienned

green onion, trimmed and thinly sliced

white sesame seeds

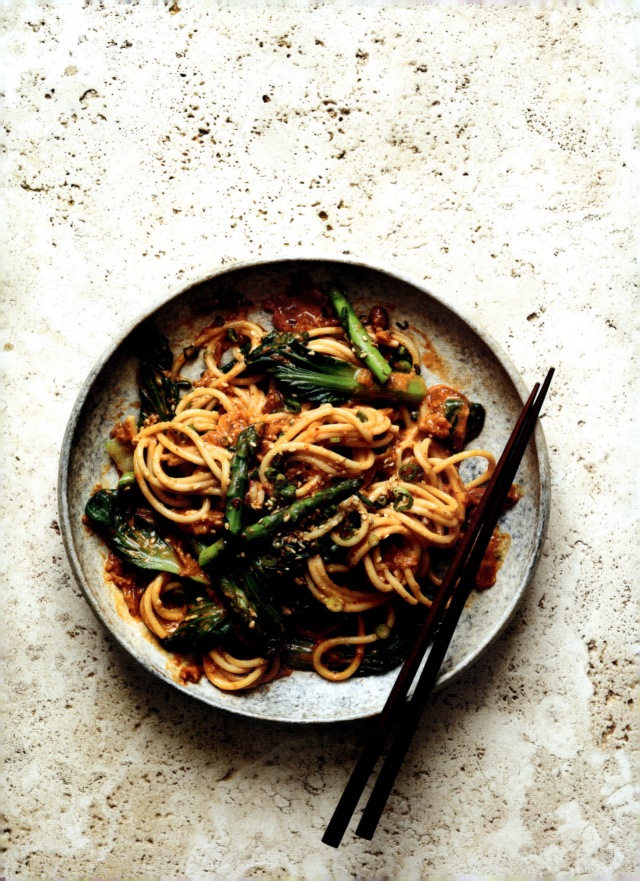

Chicken Kimchi Masala

One evening, I gave myself a challenge of making a quick curry with the ingredients I had in my pantry and fermentation larder and immediately gravitated toward kimchi, as it packs so much flavor. I wanted an Indian takeaway, so I treated the kimchi as the base paste for a South Asian–adjacent curry. And guess what—it really worked out well. It comes together quickly and has become a regular part of our weeknight repertoire. Great when you're low on time but want something flavorful and comforting.

PREP TIME: 20 MINUTES | COOK TIME: 30 MINUTES

Cut the chicken thighs into bite-size pieces. To make the marinade, blitz the kimchi in a food processor, then scrape it into a large bowl and add the yogurt, gochugaru, and garam masala. Add the chicken and mix thoroughly. Leave to marinate for around 10 minutes while you prep the next steps.

To make the paste, put all of the ingredients in a food processor and blitz to a fine paste.

Heat the oil in a large saucepan over a medium-low heat, add the paste and cook for 7–10 minutes until the liquid has reduced and the paste is jammy. Add the tomato paste and garam masala and cook for a further 2–3 minutes.

Add the marinated chicken and its marinade to the pan, turn the heat up to medium, and cook for around 7–10 minutes, stirring occasionally, until the chicken is cooked through. If the sauce starts to stick to the pan, you can add 120ml (½ cup) water.

Stir in the fish sauce and heavy cream. Depending on the kimchi you're using, the sauce may already be sweet. Otherwise, add the sugar (which really rounds out the dish) and adjust the seasoning.

Once everything is combined and warmed through, garnish with the cilantro—and additional kimchi—and serve alongside hot rice or a warmed paratha.

Serves 4

500g (1lb 2oz) skinless, boneless chicken thighs

1 tbsp vegetable oil

4 tbsp tomato paste

1 tsp garam masala

2 tsp fish sauce

150ml (½ cup plus 2 tbsp) heavy cream

1½ tsp sugar

salt and pepper

fresh cilantro to garnish

rice or paratha to serve

FOR THE MARINADE

100g (⅔ cup) kimchi, including its residual brine

150g (½ cup plus 2 tbsp) full-fat yogurt

2 tsp coarse gochugaru

2 tsp garam masala

FOR THE PASTE

1 onion, peeled and chopped

5 garlic cloves, peeled and chopped

10g (0.33oz) fresh ginger, peeled and chopped

200g (1⅓ cups) kimchi, chopped

SPECIAL EQUIPMENT: food processor

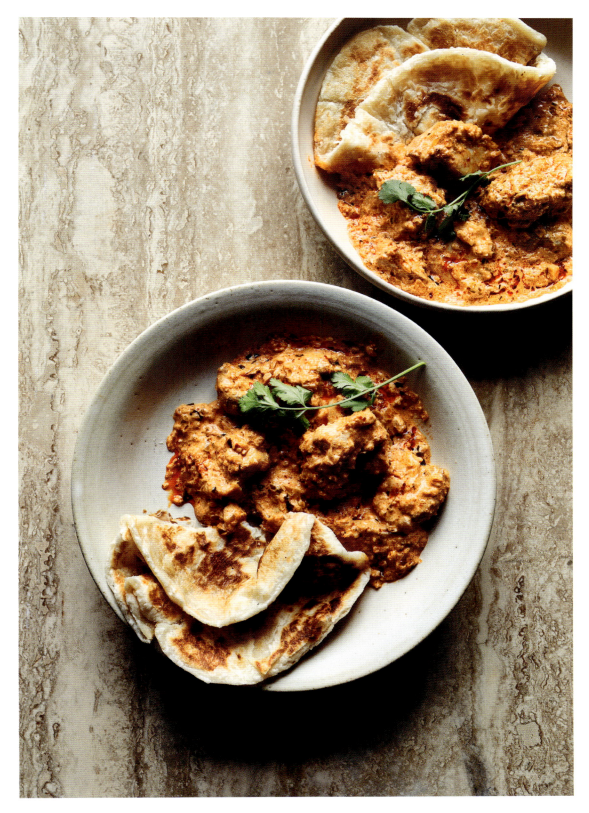

Miso-Ginger Chicken Orzo

I grew up eating okazu, a term broadly referring to a dish eaten with rice, which in my home meant a donburi, or a savory dish on top of rice, the often soy-based sauce coating the glistening grains. I grew up with two parents working full-time, so we ate variations on "stuff with rice" alongside fresh tofu and pickles (of course) several times a week. It was quick, easy, and so satisfying.

This dish is a celebration of those memories—with a bit of a Western twist—and ticks all of the boxes when I want a comforting and relatively quick meal that can be made in one pan. When I was developing this dish, I was lucky enough to have my parents in town and it was very special feeding them an evolution of a dish they themselves would make for my sister and me. Like for many of you, I'm sure, feeding others is my ultimate love language: nourishing, steeped with nostalgia, and a reminder of home, wherever that may be.

Rendering the chicken fat adds significant flavor, which is why skin-on chicken thighs are absolutely necessary for this meal. It's a forgiving dish (as weeknight meals should be), makes great leftovers, and is ultimately a gently flavored canvas for pickles and chili oil. So you really can't go wrong.

PREP TIME: 10 MINUTES | COOK TIME: 30–40 MINUTES

In a large frying pan (large enough to cook 3–4 chicken thighs in one go), heat the olive oil over a medium heat. As it's warming up, season the chicken on both sides with salt and pepper. Add the chicken, skin side down, and cook for 7 minutes until the skin releases from the pan with the help of a spatula and is golden brown. Flip the chicken thighs and cook for a further 3–5 minutes until they're cooked through. Transfer them to a plate.

Turn the heat down to low and add the onions, ginger, and garlic. Cook for 3–5 minutes until the onions have softened and then add the orzo and cook for a few more minutes, stirring continuously to allow the flavors to mingle. If the orzo starts to stick to the pan, add an extra teaspoon of olive oil.

Serves 4

6 boneless skin-on chicken thighs

1 tbsp olive oil

salt and pepper

2 white onions, peeled and finely diced

50g (1.75oz) fresh ginger, peeled and julienned

5 garlic cloves, peeled and finely chopped

200g (7oz) orzo

1½ tsp dashi powder

2 tbsp red miso

100g (¾ cup) frozen peas

Deglaze the pan by pouring in 500ml (2 cups plus 1 tablespoon) of water, stirring and scraping up the sticky bits on the bottom (flavor!). Mix in the dashi powder and miso, followed by the peas. Bring to a simmer and cook for 8–10 minutes, until the orzo is cooked through.

While this is simmering, chop the chicken thighs into bite-size pieces and place them on top of the orzo, skin side up. Pour any residual juices from the chicken back into the pan. Cook for a few more minutes—primarily to warm the chicken through—but keep an eye on the orzo as it may stick and burn.

Remove from the heat and leave to stand for 5 minutes. Garnish with green onions, a squeeze of lemon, and your choice of pickles and chili oil.

TO SERVE

3 green onions, trimmed and thinly sliced

lemon wedges

pickles

chili oil

Kimchi-Brined Fried Chicken with Gochujang Hot Honey Crumpets

When I lived on the upper west side of Manhattan, a regular treat would be going uptown to Harlem for fried chicken and waffles. Harlem was one of my favorite neighborhoods to explore, especially on Sundays when a morning excursion uptown would mean gospel music echoing from nearby churches and families in their Sunday best (and the hats!). Perhaps what made this journey much more satisfying, however, was thinking about the food that awaited me.

Korean flavors are magical with fried chicken and are increasingly popular for very good reason. This kimchi-brined fried chicken with gochujang hot honey, eaten with toasted crumpets, is my contribution to the diverse culinary traditions surrounding fried chicken. Easy yet satisfying, it does require a bit of prep, as the wet brining process needs time to fully flavor and tenderize the meat. For this reason, I generally prepare and fry more chicken than what's needed to make the most of the process (and the deep-frying). The leftovers are delicious on a rice or grain bowl, on top of a salad, or in a sandwich.

If you don't have access to crumpets you can of course eat this with English muffins, waffles, or on a large slice of toasted sourdough bread. Crumpets work perfectly to allow the gochujang hot honey to get into every nook and cranny, but regardless of your carb, be sure to be heavy handed with the gochujang hot honey. This dish pops with the freshness of kimchi, particularly my Cherry Tomato Kimchi (see page 66), where the tomatoey brine adds depth in tang and aromatics. *See photo on the next page.*

PREP TIME: 10 MINUTES + 6 hours (or overnight) brining
COOK TIME: 25 MINUTES

In a large resealable freezer bag or food-safe container with a lid, mix all of the brine ingredients and then add the chicken. I like to use a resealable bag when marinating meat so I can press out the residual air. Brine the chicken for a minimum of 6 hours or overnight in the fridge.

When you are ready to deep-fry, make the dredge by mixing all of the ingredients in a shallow bowl. Line a baking sheet or rack with paper towels.

Fill a deep cast-iron pan or wok with vegetable oil (no more than one-third full for safety) and turn the heat to high. If you're using a deep-fat fryer, heat the oil to 350°F (180°C). To check that the oil is hot enough, drop a very small amount of the dredge mixture into the oil: If it immediately rises to the top and starts to brown, it is ready.

While the oil is heating up, dredge the chicken thighs in the mixture, using some force to ensure the mixture is packed onto the chicken.

Depending on the size of your pan, cook 3–4 chicken thighs at a time—it's important to not overcrowd the pan. Leave the chicken undisturbed as it cooks. After 3–4 minutes, flip them and cook for a further 3–4 minutes, until both sides are golden brown. Immediately move them to the lined sheet or rack to absorb excess oil. Sprinkle with flaky sea salt while still warm.

To make the gochujang hot honey, put both the ingredients into a small pan and warm together until sticky and evenly combined.

To assemble the dish, toast your crumpets, slather on the gochujang hot honey, and add a piece of fried chicken and another drizzle of gochujang hot honey. Serve with kimchi on the side.

Serves 6

6 skinless, boneless chicken thighs

vegetable oil for deep-frying

flaky sea salt

6 crumpets (or English muffins, waffles, or sourdough bread slices)

kimchi to serve

FOR THE BRINE

100ml (¼ cup plus 3 tbsp) kimchi brine

200ml (¾ cup plus 1 tbsp) buttermilk (or use all kimchi brine if you have it)

1 medium egg

2 tbsp fish sauce

TO DREDGE

100g (¾ cup plus 1 tbsp) all-purpose flour

4 tbsp cornstarch

1 tsp baking powder

1 tsp salt

35g (¼ cup) black and white sesame seeds

FOR THE GOCHUJANG HOT HONEY

100ml (¼ cup plus 3 tbsp) clear honey

160g (½ cup plus 1 tbsp) gochujang

SPECIAL EQUIPMENT: deep-fat fryer (optional)

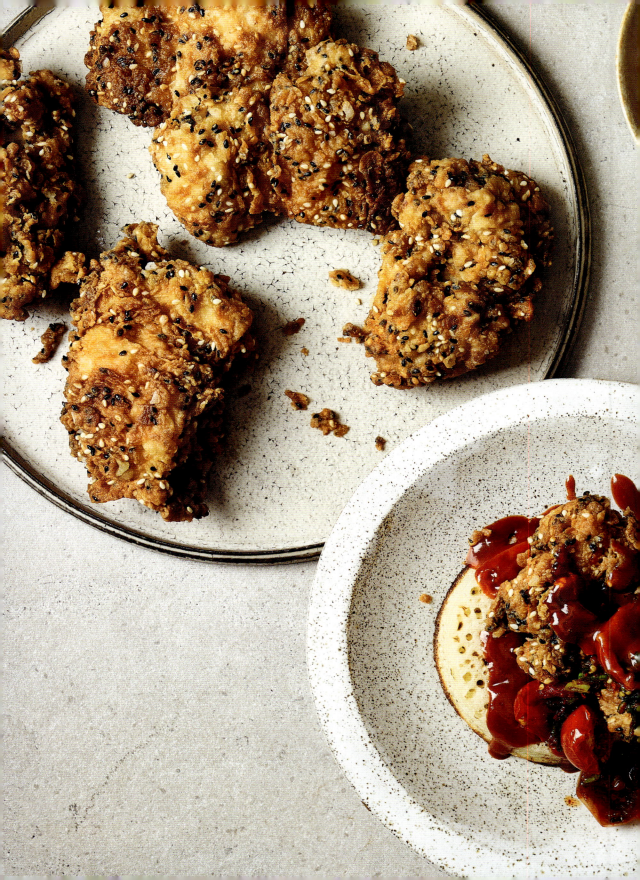

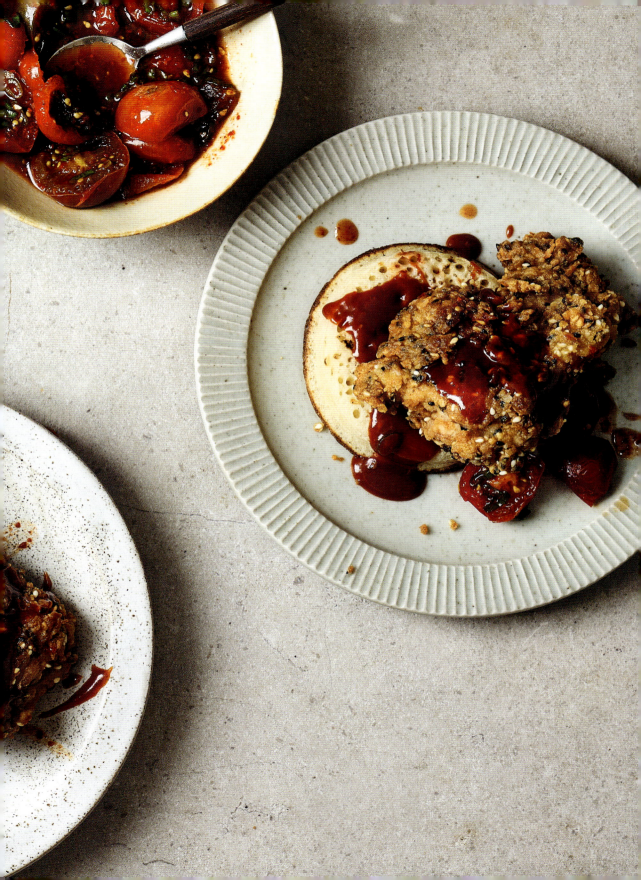

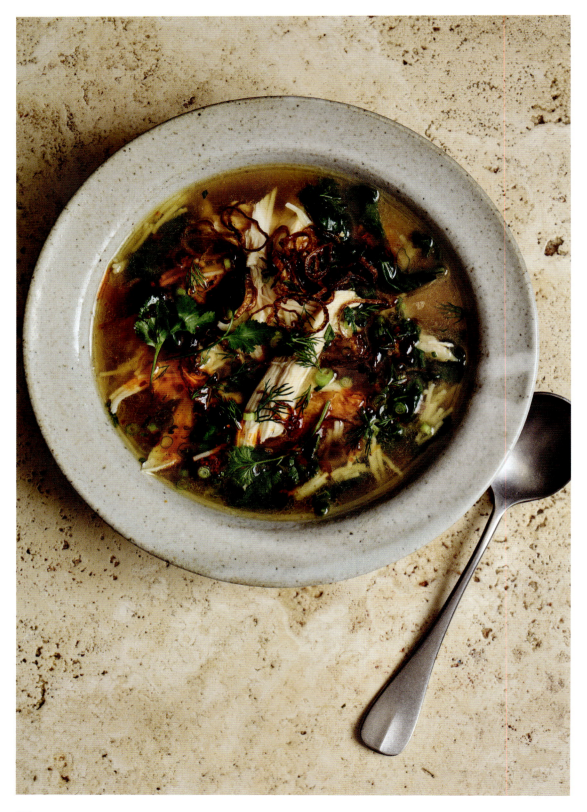

Leftover (Sunday) Roast Chicken Miso Noodle Soup

One of the British culinary traditions I've adopted is the glorious Sunday roast. In my home, this usually takes the form of a roast chicken, roast potatoes, and sautéed or steamed greens, with a selection of pickles and ferments to offset what can be a rather heavy meal.

As Monday rolls around, I like to repurpose leftovers in a different but equally satisfying way. Regardless of how much chicken is left over from the night before, the chicken bones are the building blocks for a flavor-packed meal which reduces kitchen waste and also acts as a template for endless customization. When making stock, more is more, so feel free to add other ingredients to those suggested below if you're keen to use up vegetables. Also remember that this is a template—you can make a great stock even if you're missing one of the ingredients. The chicken carcass is non-negotiable, but the stock can easily be made with leftover bones from chicken thighs or drumsticks.

Make the stock on Sunday evening so you can easily put this together in under 20 minutes when you come home from work.

This recipe (surprisingly!) can easily be made vegan by swapping in vegetable broth or vegetarian kombu seaweed broth and tofu.

PREP TIME: 20 MINUTES | COOK TIME: 2–3 HOURS

First make the stock. Put all of the ingredients into a heavy-bottomed pot and cover with about 1.5 liters (1.5 quarts) of water, so all of the ingredients are entirely submerged. Bring to a boil and then reduce to a simmer for 2–3 hours. As it cooks, the flavors will intensify. You may need to skim off any residue that accumulates on the surface. Add more water if it reduces too much. Strain the stock and it's ready to use. The stock will keep for a few days in the fridge or up to 2 months in the freezer.

Ingredients and recipe continue on the next page

Serves 4–6

FOR THE STOCK

1 chicken carcass, all meat removed

1 white onion, peeled and cut in half

1 celery stick, cut into thirds

1 carrot, cut in half (peel included)

3 garlic cloves (left in their skin)

1 piece of fresh ginger

handful of black peppercorns

To make the soup, bring a small pot of water to a boil. Add the vermicelli to a bowl, cover with the boiling water, and let soak for 7 minutes.

If necessary, bring the stock back to a gentle simmer. Dissolve the miso in the stock: The best way to do this is to put the miso in a large ladle with some of the warm liquid and mix to ensure there are no large clumps of miso.

Add the leftover vegetables to the soup to warm them through. Once the noodles are ready, it's plating time!

Layer the noodles into warmed bowls, then ladle in the broth. Top with the vegetables and leftover chicken. The chicken will warm up as you add the finishing touches: herbs, sliced green onions, a generous sprinkle of sesame seeds, crispy fried shallots, kimchi sprinkles for a hot and sour bite, if desired, lime for acidity, and chili oil to seal the deal.

FOR THE SOUP

vermicelli noodles (about 30g/1oz per person)

2 tbsp red miso

leftover green vegetables, such as spring greens, spinach, or brussels sprouts (best if they are not heavily seasoned or spiced and ideally steamed, roasted, or sautéed)

leftover roast chicken, shredded or cut into bite-size pieces

TO SERVE

fresh herbs, such as cilantro or dill

green onions, thinly sliced

sesame seeds

crispy fried shallots

Kimchi Sprinkles (see page 76) (optional)

1 lime, cut into quarters

chili oil

Bacon, Leek & Kimchi Quiche

Without much effort, you'll quickly learn that pork, alliums, kimchi, and cheese are a phenomenal combination. And even better against a custardy base and flaky homemade pastry. You know those recipes that are so associated with home? That is what I want this to be for my family.

I find something incredibly elegant and special about a quiche. It is a multi-step process, so I reserve this dish for when I have a lazy weekend for a cooking project. You can of course use store-bought shortcrust pastry, but a homemade version is really worth the effort (and then you can brag about it). It can even be made a day or two in advance. While you can reheat it, cold, straight-from-the-fridge quiche has a special place in my heart. *See photo on the next page.*

PREP TIME: 30 MINUTES + chilling time | COOK TIME: 1 HOUR

MAINS

First make the pastry: Put the flour, salt, and butter into a food processor and blitz to the consistency of bread crumbs. Slowly add 65ml (¼ cup plus 1 teaspoon) cold water while pulsing the food processor, until a rough ball of dough has formed. If you don't have a food processor, sift the flour and salt into a mixing bowl, add the cubed butter, and rub into the flour using your fingertips until the mixture resembles bread crumbs. Sprinkle the water into the bowl and mix gently to create a dough. Wrap the dough tightly in plastic wrap or parchment paper and move to the fridge for at least 1 hour.

Heat a frying pan over a medium heat and cook the bacon for 3–5 minutes until some of the fat has rendered. Add the vegetable oil, followed by the sliced leek and kimchi, and cook for 7–9 minutes until everything is cooked through and jammy. Set aside.

Dust your work surface with flour. Roll out the pastry to a disc around 12cm (5in) larger than your tart pan (see the next page). Lay the pastry in the pan and press it down against the base and edges. Prick the base with a fork before returning it to the fridge for 15 minutes.

Special equipment list and recipe continue on the next page

Serves 6–8

12 slices of dry-cured streaky bacon (about 225g/8oz), roughly chopped into small pieces

1 tsp vegetable oil

1 small-medium leek (100g/3.5oz), trimmed, washed, and sliced

175g (1¼ cups) kimchi, chopped

4 medium eggs

200ml (¾ cup plus 1 tbsp) whole milk

100g (1 cup) cheddar, grated and divided into two equal parts

2 green onions, thinly sliced

FOR THE PASTRY

185g (1½ cups) all-purpose flour, plus extra for dusting

1 tsp salt

100g (7 tbsp) cold unsalted butter, cubed

Put a baking sheet into the oven and preheat to 425°F (220°C).

In order to prevent a soggy bottom on your quiche, blind bake the pastry. To do this, line the pastry case with parchment paper, fill it with dried beans, raw rice, or ceramic baking beans, and place it on the heated baking sheet. Bake for 15 minutes, then remove the paper and weights and bake for a further 5 minutes, until the pastry is a light brown color.

Remove from the oven and trim any overhanging pastry. Turn the heat down to 400°F (200°C).

In a jug, whisk together the eggs and milk.

Scatter the bacon and kimchi mixture over the cooked pastry, followed by half of the grated cheese, and then pour in the egg mixture. Scatter over the remaining cheese and the sliced green onions and bake for 25–30 minutes until the pastry is golden, the filling is set, and the cheese is browning on top.

Let the quiche cool for 15–20 minutes before digging in. However, I generally prefer a cold quiche, so be excited for the leftovers!

SPECIAL EQUIPMENT: 20-cm (8-in) tart pan with removable bottom; food processor (optional)

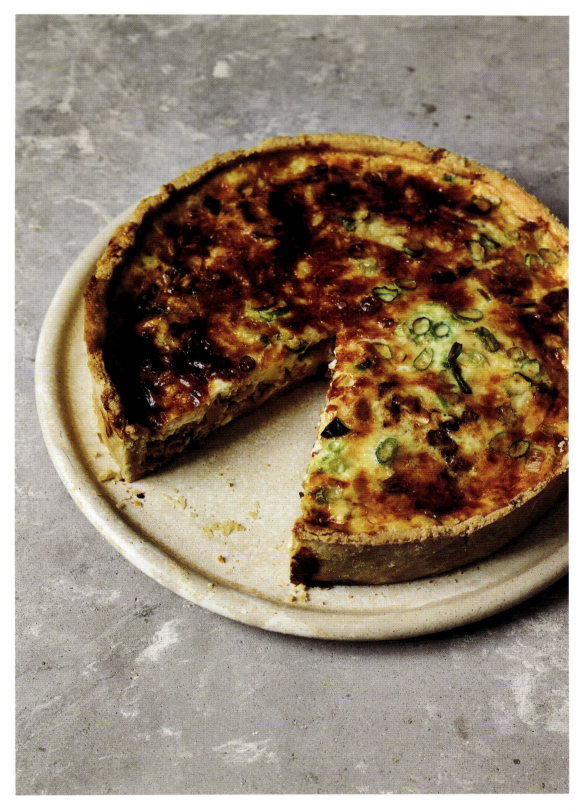

Nasu Dengaku Moussaka

This is a combination of two of my favorite dishes from very different parts of the world: nasu dengaku, eggplant roasted with a sweet miso sauce; and moussaka, a hearty baked eggplant and lamb dish. This version plays with those two flavor profiles, leaning more heavily into the Japanese dengaku notes of ginger, garlic, and miso, but connected to the moussaka with the lamb, tomato paste, and a delicious nutmeg béchamel. As with most moussaka, the recipe may appear to be a lot of work, but the three elements (or the entire moussaka) can be made ahead of time and assembled and baked when needed. If you spend a lazy weekend cooking, make an activity of it with your favorite music and a glass of wine.

This makes a comforting meal alongside a fresh herb and citrus salad, such as my Bitter Greens Salad with Pickled Pear Vinaigrette (see page 186).

You can use a different size of oven-safe dish but may need to adjust the timing slightly. Generally, keep an eye on it when baking—each oven is different. *See photos on the next page.*

PREP TIME: 45 MINUTES | COOK TIME: 1 HOUR 15 MINUTES

Preheat the oven to 400°F (200°C). Line two large baking sheets with parchment paper.

While the oven is warming up, lightly salt the sliced eggplants and set aside for 15–20 minutes.

Dab any excess water from the eggplants with a paper towel. Put them into a large bowl and drizzle with 3 tablespoons of the olive oil; I use my hands to ensure the eggplant is evenly coated. It may not seem like enough oil but remember that the eggplant will be cooked further in the moussaka. Lay the eggplant in a single layer on the lined baking sheets and bake for 15–20 minutes until cooked through and fork tender. Remove from the oven and leave to cool.

While the eggplant is in the oven, start on the lamb.

Serves 8

- 3 large eggplants, about 300g (10.5oz) each, cut into roughly 5-mm (¼-in) slices
- salt and pepper
- 90ml (¼ cup plus 2 tbsp) olive oil
- 1kg (2.25lbs) ground lamb
- 2 onions, peeled and finely chopped
- 20g (0.75oz) finely chopped fresh ginger
- 20g (0.75oz) finely chopped garlic
- 225ml (¾ cup plus 3 tbsp) dry vermouth, white wine, or sake (or water)
- 3 tbsp tomato paste
- 3 tbsp red miso
- 1 tbsp sugar

In a large heavy-bottomed frying pan over a medium heat, add the remaining 3 tablespoons of olive oil and the ground lamb. Cook for 8–10 minutes, stirring regularly to break up any large clumps of meat, until all of the liquid has cooked off. Add the onions, ginger, and garlic and cook for 2–3 minutes.

Deglaze the pan by pouring in the vermouth. Add the tomato paste, red miso, sugar, and 225ml (¾ cup plus 3 tablespoons) of water and bring to a simmer; cook for 10–15 minutes, stirring occasionally, until the sauce has thickened.

During this time, make the béchamel. Melt the butter in a saucepan over a medium heat. Once fully melted, stir in the flour and cook for 1–2 minutes until the color slightly deepens. Gradually add the milk, whisking gently. As the milk cooks with the flour and butter, the béchamel will start to thicken. Continue to whisk until it's smooth and season with grated nutmeg. Set aside to cool slightly; it will thicken as it cools.

Spread half the lamb mixture into your oven-safe dish, followed by a layer of half the eggplant slices. Repeat the layers. Carefully pour the béchamel over the final eggplant layer and smooth it over. Bake for 30–45 minutes until the béchamel has browned. Leave to cool for 10–15 minutes before digging in. If you like, serve up with Bitter Greens Salad with Pickled Pear Vinaigrette (see page 186).

Once cooled, the moussaka can be frozen.

FOR THE BÉCHAMEL

50g (4 tbsp) unsalted butter

50g (¼ cup plus 2 tbsp) all-purpose flour

450ml (1¾ cups plus 2 tbsp) whole milk

½ nutmeg, grated

SPECIAL EQUIPMENT: 23 x 33-cm (9 x 13-in) oven-safe dish

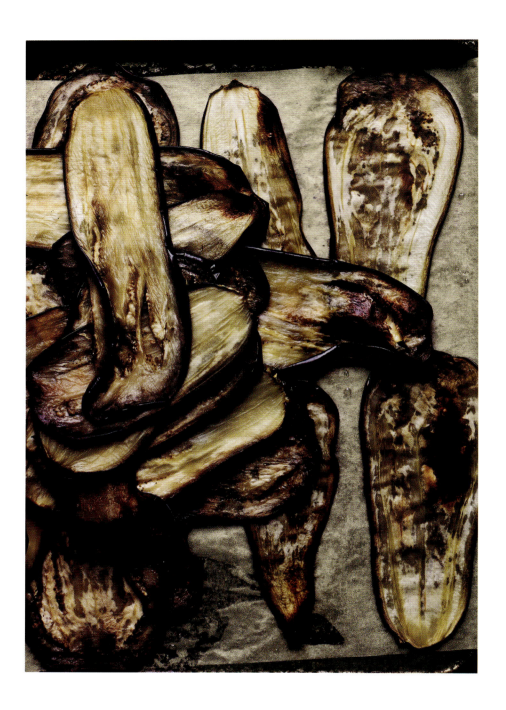

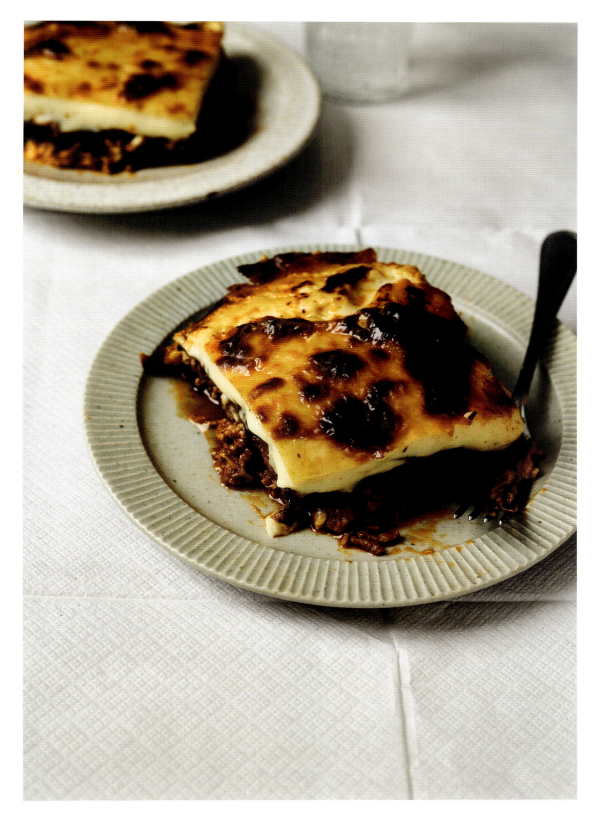

Kraut & Sausage Soup with Sour Cream & Parsley

This one-pot meal is hearty! It's packed full of greens, sausage, and beans and allows sauerkraut—the star of the dish—to really shine. Using different varieties of sauerkraut yields different soups (one of the best things about this recipe!)—which is why the other ingredients are fairly simple, with no additional spices or herbs. Instead, you let the sauerkraut do the heavy lifting. It's also very easy to adapt—throw in spinach, kale, celery, frozen mixed vegetables ... you name it.

Cooking sauerkraut not only adds flavor with a subtle sourness to the soup, but it is also texturally exciting, the fermented shredded vegetables melting into each bite. This soup unintentionally resembles the sauerkraut soups common in Eastern Europe, which were a product of frugality and accessibility, as the cold winter months meant a reliance on sauerkraut. It was, coincidentally, a meal born in my home kitchen from using pantry staples at the end of the month combined with intuition to put together a rather delicious and warming soup.

PREP TIME: 10 MINUTES | COOK TIME: 45 MINUTES

Heat a large heavy-bottomed pan over a medium heat with 1 tablespoon of the olive oil. If using sausages, use a sharp knife to slit the sausage casings and remove the meat. Cook the sausage meat for 5–7 minutes, breaking it up into chunks, until nicely browned. Transfer the meat to a bowl.

Add another tablespoon of oil to the pan and fry the onion for 4–5 minutes, then add the garlic and cook for 1–2 minutes. Add the leeks and cook for a further 5–7 minutes, stirring continuously.

Add the beans, sauerkraut, and cooked sausage to the pan, followed by the chicken stock. Bring to a boil, then reduce the heat to a simmer and cook for 15–20 minutes. Season with salt and pepper.

Serve in warmed bowls with a squeeze of lemon juice, a dollop of sour cream, and some chopped parsley. I also rather like it with a few dashes of Everyday Hot Sauce (see page 45).

Serves 4–6

2 tbsp olive oil

400g (14oz) sausage meat (or the meat from 6 sausages)

1 onion, peeled and finely chopped

2 garlic cloves, peeled and finely chopped

200g (7oz) leeks, quartered, washed and roughly chopped

500g (3 cups) cooked beans, such as kidney, black, or pinto, drained

300g (2 cups) sauerkraut, including its residual brine

1.4 liters (1.4 quarts) chicken stock

salt and pepper

lemon wedges, sour cream, and chopped fresh parsley to garnish

Miso Short Rib Birria Tacos with Kimchi Guacamole & Umami Slaw

There is nothing traditional nor authentic about this recipe: It is an ode to the Tex-Mex Korean fusion which blew my mind when I visited California as a teenager. As I've grown up away from my family and home, I've always been fascinated by how food evolves as a function of time and place; some of the best dishes I've had in my life are a result of the confluence of people and cultures, with food being the best way to celebrate these interactions.

The short ribs take some time to cook but leave you with plenty of leftovers, so treat this as a weekend project or a way to batch-prep meals for the coming week. Once the short ribs are done, the meat can easily be reheated (or frozen) for a quick weeknight dinner where all you'll need to do is make the sides and assemble. This recipe should have more than enough meat for eight 15-cm (6-in) tacos. Leftovers are perfect for a rice or grain bowl, to which the guacamole and slaw make great accompaniments. *See photo on the next page.*

PREP TIME: 30 MINUTES | COOK TIME: 4 HOURS 50 MINUTES

Preheat the oven to 350°F (180°C).

Season the short ribs with salt and pepper. Heat a large stovetop-safe casserole dish or Dutch oven over a medium heat, add 1 tablespoon of oil, and brown the ribs; take time to ensure they are browned on all sides.

Add 2 liters (2 quarts) of water and all of the braising liquid ingredients. Bring to a boil, then cover and cook in the oven for around 4 hours. Check every 30 minutes to ensure the short ribs are submerged, flipping them after around 2 hours.

Once the meat is fork tender and falling from the bones, lift out the meat and shred it with two forks.

Put the casserole dish over a low heat and simmer until the braising liquid reduces by half or three quarters to make a rich thick sauce.

Ingredients and recipe continue on the next page

Serves 4–6

1kg (2.25lbs) beef short ribs

salt and pepper

FOR THE BRAISING LIQUID

1 beef stock cube

140g (½ cup) red miso

60ml (¼ cup) mirin

50g (¼ cup) brown sugar

40g (1.5oz) fresh ginger, peeled and sliced

10 garlic cloves, peeled and left whole

1 tbsp sriracha or similar hot sauce

1 tsp freshly cracked black pepper

You can make the guacamole and cabbage slaw while the ribs are in the oven. For the guacamole, mash the avocado flesh in a bowl with lemon juice to taste. Stir in the kimchi and season liberally with salt and pepper.

For the slaw, shred the cabbage finely, using a mandoline or a sharp knife. Put it into a bowl and mix in the yogurt, white miso, lemon zest, and juice.

To serve, heat a frying pan over a medium heat with 1 teaspoon of vegetable oil. Dip a tortilla in the reduced braising liquid and then carefully lower it into the hot pan. As it sizzles, layer on crumbled feta, shredded meat, and cilantro, but do not put too many ingredients in the taco as you will be folding it in half. Cook for 3–5 minutes and remove to a baking sheet. Transfer to the oven to keep warm while you cook the remaining tacos. Serve immediately, with the guacamole and slaw, garnished with the Quick-Pickled Kombucha Chiles.

FOR THE KIMCHI GUACAMOLE

2 ripe avocados

1–2 tsp lemon juice

100g (⅔ cup) kimchi, finely chopped

salt and pepper

FOR THE SLAW

¼ red cabbage (about 225g/8oz)

3 tbsp full-fat yogurt

1 tbsp white miso

zest of 1 lemon and juice of ½ lemon

TO SERVE

1 tbsp vegetable oil, plus 1 tsp

flour tortillas, 15cm (6in) in diameter

200g (¾ cup) feta, crumbled

handful of fresh cilantro, roughly chopped

Quick-Pickled Kombucha Chiles (see page 112) or Quick-Pickled Red Onions (see page 114)

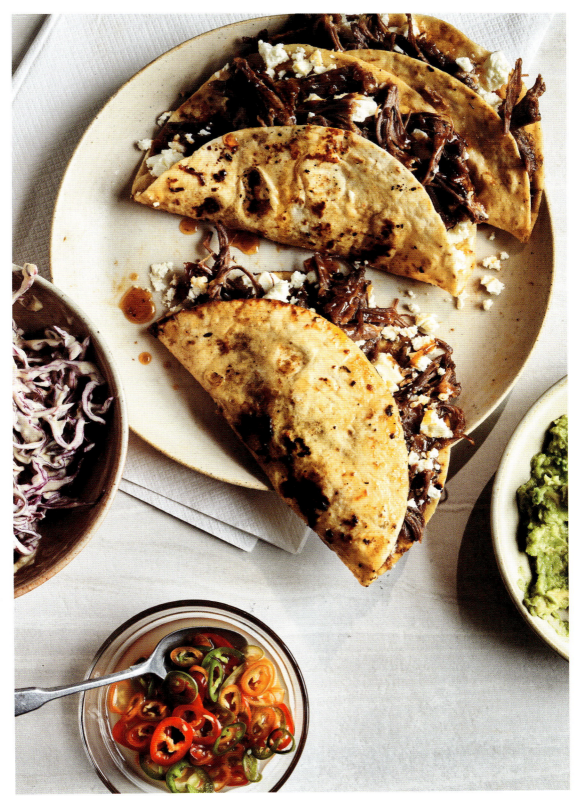

DESSERTS

Miso Praline Sesame Pecans

Which do you prefer: pumpkin pie or pecan pie? As an American, I'm often asked this question as Thanksgiving approaches. I've always jumped to pumpkin pie, as it is usually less cloyingly sweet than the pecan pies that graced our Thanksgiving table. Admittedly my sweet tooth has developed as I've gotten older, but I naturally gravitate toward desserts that aren't too sweet. Many of my Asian readers may relate to this: The best compliment many desserts can receive from an elder is that it's "not too sweet." So here's my "not too sweet" savory miso and sesame praline pecans: an homage to my Japanese American Thanksgiving table and the perfect snacking treat.

This recipe is fairly adjustable: Add a pinch of flaky sea salt to the mix if you like it more savory or use a 50:50 blend of pecans and walnuts. This makes a really easy (and delicious) gift.

PREP TIME: 10 MINUTES | COOK TIME: 45–60 MINUTES

Makes 400g (14oz)

1 egg white
1 tbsp plus 1½ tsp white miso
400g (4 cups) pecan halves
1 tbsp black sesame seeds
1 tbsp white sesame seeds
100g (½ cup) granulated sugar
100g (½ cup) light brown sugar

Preheat the oven to 285°F (140°C) and line a baking sheet with parchment paper.
  In a small mixing bowl, whisk the egg white until frothy and the color has changed to white—you do not need soft peaks. In another small bowl, mix the miso with 1 tablespoon of water until you have a thin paste, then add the diluted miso to the egg white and fold until combined.
  Add the pecans and sesame seeds and mix until they are coated with the mixture, then add both types of sugar and mix until combined.
  Spread the pecans in a single layer on the lined baking sheet and bake for 45–60 minutes, stirring every 15–20 minutes.
  Leave to cool to room temperature before enjoying. Keep in an airtight container for up to 1 month.

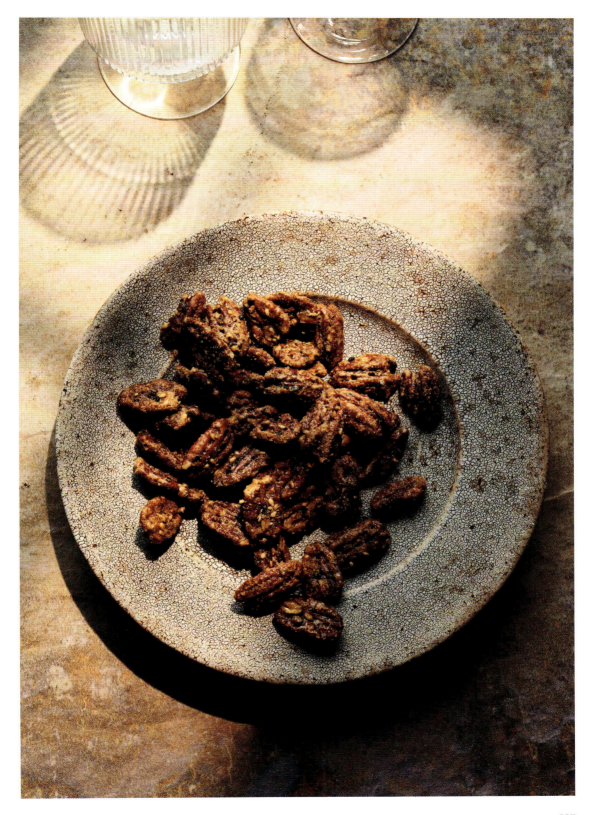

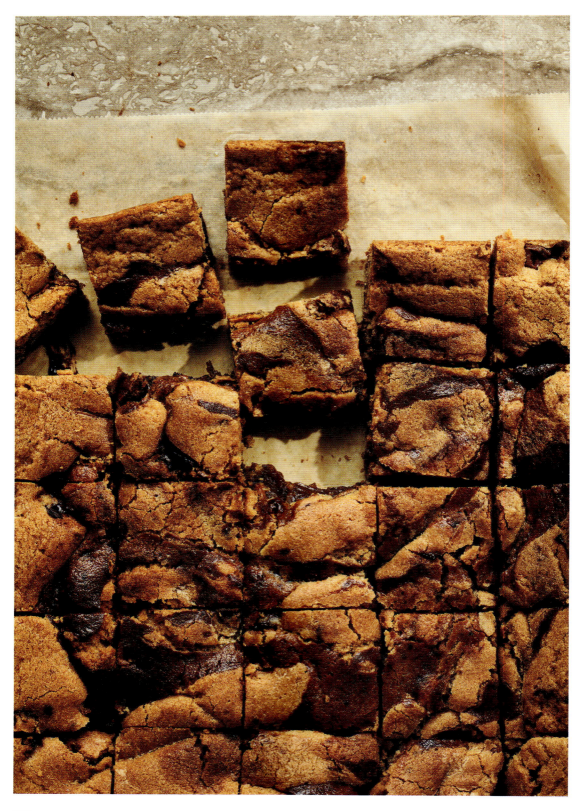

Miso Tahini Chocolate Chip Blondies

My sister is an incredible baker with a penchant for bar cookies and particularly blondies. Whenever we were all home for the holidays, she would bake up a storm, including ten varieties of perfectly round bite-size cookies. These would always require my grandmother's approval for our New Year's cookie trays, a baking task which once sat entirely with her. Toward the end of my grandmother's life my sister would still look for that approval with each cookie recipe perfected: seeing how many cookies my very small grandmother would eat and, in her last New Year with us, give a quiet nod and smile with each bite.

I've never been much of a baker, as I found it too scientific; I do appreciate the irony of this now, with my passion for fermentation. But these blondies are my contribution to the symbolic New Year's cookie tray. And I think my grandmother would have liked them—a good balance of sweet and savory ("not too sweet"), slight nuttiness from the tahini, and, of course, chocolate chips.

PREP TIME: 15 MINUTES | COOK TIME: 35 MINUTES

Preheat the oven to 375°F (190°C). Butter the cake pan and line with parchment paper.

In a large mixing bowl, beat the butter with both types of sugar until fully combined and airy. If using an electric mixer at medium-high speed, this should take 3–5 minutes. Then reduce the speed to low and beat in the vanilla and eggs, followed by the flour and baking soda. Fold in the chocolate chips. Scrape the batter into the prepared pan and smooth over the top.

Make the tahini topping in a small mixing bowl, mixing all of the ingredients together until fully combined. The mixture will be rather thick, so dollop small amounts of it on top of the blondie batter: It will melt as it bakes.

Bake for around 35 minutes. You'll know it's done when the sides of the bake begin to pull away from the pan and the center is firm to the touch. Leave to cool completely in the pan before cutting into squares.

Keep in an airtight container for 3–5 days.

Makes 25 squares

- **225g (1 cup) unsalted butter, softened, at room temperature, plus extra for greasing**
- **160g (¾ cup plus 1 tbsp) light brown sugar**
- **125g (½ cup plus 2 tbsp) granulated sugar**
- **1 tsp vanilla extract**
- **2 medium eggs**
- **240g (2 cups) all-purpose flour**
- **1 tsp baking soda**
- **200g (1¼ cups) chocolate chips (dark or milk)**

FOR THE TAHINI TOPPING

- **80g (⅓ cup) tahini**
- **50g (¼ cup) light brown sugar**
- **1 tbsp white miso**

SPECIAL EQUIPMENT: 23-cm (9-in) square cake pan; electric mixer (optional)

Citrus Kombucha Cookies

It's funny how a recipe can immediately transport you to a time and place and this is exactly what happened here. It started with an idea: How can I use one preserved ingredient in different forms to create a dish? My kombucha citrus syrup came to mind as it has two elements to it: the delicious syrup and the preserved and almost candied citrus slices. When puréed, the preserved citrus becomes jammy and tart—perhaps this could work well in a cookie batter, I thought. And the syrup? The base of a glaze.

And with the first bite, I was transported back to when I used to sit around the dining room table after school, green tea in hand, enjoying the soft lemon moon-shaped cookies my mom would occasionally bring home after work. These, like those, are a bit cakey, soft, and tempting.

PREP TIME: 30 MINUTES + 15 minutes chilling
COOK TIME: 10–15 MINUTES

Put the preserved citrus slices in a food processor and blitz to a purée.

In a large mixing bowl, beat the butter and brown sugar until fully combined and airy. If using an electric mixer at medium-high speed, this should take 3–5 minutes. Mix in the egg and puréed citrus, then fold in the flour, baking powder, and salt. Move the bowl to the fridge for 15 minutes to firm up slightly. Preheat the oven to 400°F (200°C).

Line a baking sheet with parchment paper and drop tablespoonfuls of the mixture onto the baking sheet, aiming to make 18 cookies. While these cookies will not spread too much, ensure they're spread out evenly. Bake for 10–15 minutes until cooked through. Allow to cool slightly for a few minutes, then transfer to a wire rack and leave to cool completely.

While they cool, make the glaze by whisking together the icing sugar and kombucha citrus syrup.

Once the cookies are cold, dunk them into the glaze and transfer to a lined baking sheet to set. Keep in an airtight container for up to 5 days.

Makes 16–18 cookies

- 150g (5oz) drained citrus slices from Kombucha Citrus Syrup (see page 138)
- 60g (4½ tbsp) unsalted butter, softened, at room temperature
- 120g (½ cup plus 1 tbsp) light brown sugar
- 1 medium egg
- 190g (heaping 1½ cups) all-purpose flour
- ¼ tsp baking powder
- ¼ tsp salt

FOR THE GLAZE

- 40g (¼ cup plus 1 tbsp) confectioners' sugar
- 3–4 tbsp Kombucha Citrus Syrup (see page 138)

SPECIAL EQUIPMENT: food processor; electric mixer (optional)

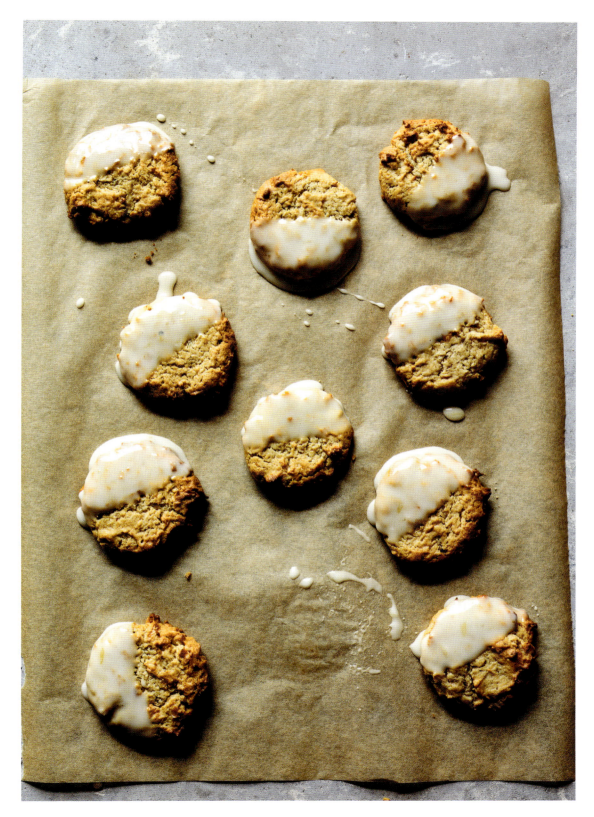

Preserved Rhubarb & Mixed Berry Pound Cake

My mom is known within the family for her pound cake. She'd bring it to countless family events and it soon became a known (and expected) treat among my college friends as she'd often send them in care packages. My mom would actually freeze them once cooled and by the time they arrived at my dorm across the country, they were ready to eat.

This one is incredibly straightforward and reliable and is truly the definition of a "one-step everyday cake"—as my mom says, you simply mix all of the ingredients together and bake! This is my riff on this coveted recipe.

The rhubarb is the star of this pound cake, with the mixed berry cheong adding extra flavor (as well as a pretty marbled effect). If you you are making only one cheong for this recipe, however, go with the rhubarb and omit the mixed berry cheong.

PREP TIME: 15 MINUTES | COOK TIME: 1 HOUR 10 MINUTES

Preheat the oven to 350°F (180°C). Butter and flour a 900-g (2-lb) loaf pan.

Put all of the ingredients (except the rhubarb and the berry cheong) into a large bowl (or electric mixer) and mix until you have a smooth and slightly thick batter. Stir in the preserved rhubarb.

Pour the batter into the prepared pan and spread evenly. Dollop the berry cheong on top of the cake and use a fork to swirl a marbled pattern.

Bake for around 1 hour 10 minutes until golden brown. To check the cake is fully baked, insert a wooden skewer into the center—if it pulls out clean, the cake is good to go. If the batter clings to the skewer, bake for a few more minutes.

Remove from the oven and leave to cool completely. Serve decorated with the extra preserved rhubarb and syrup.

This cake keeps rather well and is even better on the second day. However, it's best eaten within a week. It also freezes well.

Makes one 900-g (2-lb) loaf cake

- 200g (1½ cups plus 1 tbsp) all-purpose flour, plus extra for dusting
- 200g (1 cup) sugar
- ¼ tsp baking soda
- ¼ tsp salt
- 2 medium eggs
- 1 tsp vanilla extract
- 130g (½ cup plus 1 tbsp) unsalted butter, softened, at room temperature, plus extra for greasing
- 130g (½ cup) full-fat Greek-style yogurt
- 150g (5oz) preserved rhubarb from Rhubarb Cheong (see page 144), plus extra fruit and syrup to decorate
- 2–3 tbsp Mixed Berry Cheong (see page 144)

SPECIAL EQUIPMENT: 900-g (2-lb) loaf pan; electric mixer (optional)

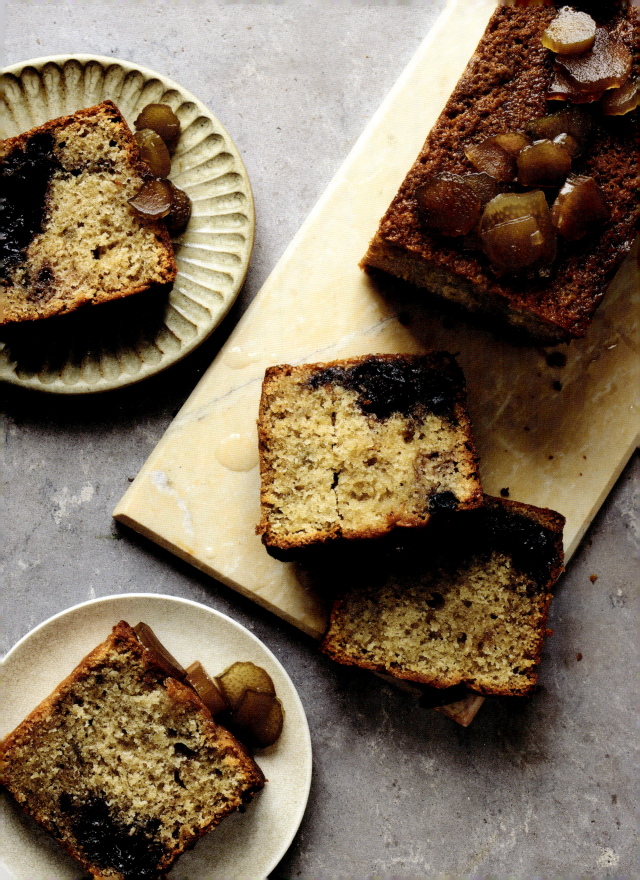

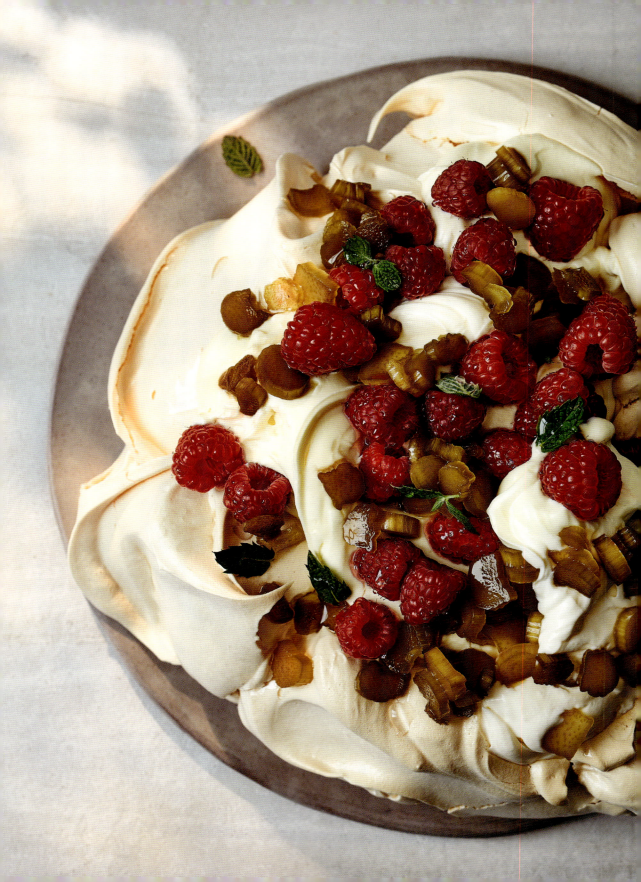

Rhubarb Cheong Pavlova

As much as I love pavlovas, and their cousin, the Eton mess, they can lean sweet. After all, you are layering sweet on sweet: a pillowy meringue, whipped cream (often sweetened), and ripe fruit (sometimes macerated with sugar to provide saucy interest).

And with this last element, enter the magic of preservation: A rhubarb cheong brings the dish together. Even better with thick, creamy yogurt, a tart flavor that offsets the sweetness of this dessert beautifully. This will work with all fruit-forward varieties of cheong: Some of my favorites are raspberry, stone fruit, and cherry. Get creative with the fresh fruit you use to adorn the pavlova. Mint is a non-negotiable for me—it adds a verdant note of freshness, which is exactly what you need at the end of a meal.

PREP TIME: 20 MINUTES
COOK TIME: 1 HOUR + 45–60 minutes cooling

Preheat the oven to 325°F (160°C). Line a baking sheet with parchment paper.

Whisk the egg whites in a bowl to stiff peaks. Using an electric hand mixer will make this much easier. Add the sugar gradually, folding it in until combined, then stir in the vinegar and cornstarch.

Spoon the meringue mixture onto the baking sheet in a circular shape around 28cm (11in) wide, building up the sides slightly higher than the center. Bake for 1 hour. Turn off the oven and let the meringue cool in the oven.

To assemble the pavlova, put the meringue on a serving dish. Whip the cream until stiff and gently mix in the yogurt. Dollop this in the center of the meringue, followed by the fresh raspberries, the cheong-preserved rhubarb, and a generous drizzle of the rhubarb cheong syrup. Finish with a scattering of mint leaves.

Serves 6–8

160ml (⅔ cup) egg whites (4–5 eggs, depending on size); yolks can be frozen or used in the Miso Caesar Dressing (see page 194)

200g (1 cup) sugar

1 tsp white wine vinegar

1 tsp cornstarch

200ml (¾ cup plus 1 tbsp) heavy cream

300g (1¼ cups) full-fat yogurt

300g (2½ cups) fresh raspberries

4–5 tbsp Rhubarb Cheong (see page 144), both syrup and preserved rhubarb

10–15 fresh mint leaves

SPECIAL EQUIPMENT: electric hand mixer (optional)

Cut Fruit with Kombucha Citrus Syrup & Kimchi Sprinkles

This is less a recipe than it is a love letter to all of the families who show their love through cut fruit. Cut or peeled fruit was a mainstay in our home, and in my grandparents' homes: I remember my grandfather silently offering a small dish of cut apple and persimmon as I watched TV in their living room, or a platter of fruit just appearing as if by magic.

Most fruit will work here. I prefer harder fruit, such as apples and pears, but this will also work well with oranges, watermelon, and pineapple. In many cultures, fruit is eaten with chili powder; here, I balance the heat and tang of the kimchi sprinkles with the kombucha citrus syrup.

PREP TIME: 5 MINUTES

Cut your fruit, drizzle the kombucha citrus syrup over it, then top with kimchi sprinkles. Enjoy immediately.

fresh fruit
Kombucha Citrus Syrup (see page 138)
Kimchi Sprinkles (see page 76)

Date & Miso Sticky Toffee Crêpe Cake

For those of you who aren't bakers, I present the ultimate dinner-party dessert showstopper. A lot of work goes into a crêpe cake, but the actual process is quite simple. And what a glorious feeling when your fork glides through the layers of cream, date-flavored crêpes, and miso sticky toffee.

The key to crêpe making is resilience: Your first crêpe may be discouraging, but by the second one you should be more at ease when it comes to controlling the heat of the pan. Confidence will grow as you learn to anticipate that exact second when the crêpe starts to crisp along the edges and the center bubbles up with steam. The crêpes need to cool before layering with the cream, and the sauce is best when cooled to room temperature. The last thing anyone wants is a melting crêpe cake. All elements of the crêpe cake can—and should—be made in advance and then assembled before a meal.

I am not saying this is a replacement for sticky toffee pudding, by far one of my favorite British desserts; however, it is a gorgeous alternative. The white miso offers a subtle umami saltiness to the sticky toffee sauce and, best yet, no need to turn on the oven! *See photo on the next page.*

PREP TIME: 20 MINUTES + chilling | COOK TIME: 40–50 MINUTES

To make the crêpe batter, put the milk and dates in a blender or food processor and blitz until completely smooth. Add the eggs and butter and blend to incorporate, then add the flour and cornstarch and blitz to a smooth batter. Cover and move to the fridge for around 45 minutes to relax the gluten.

While the batter is resting, make the sauce. Put all of the ingredients (see next page) in a small pan over a low heat and stir until thick and glossy. Set aside and leave to cool completely.

Serves 12+

FOR THE CRÊPE BATTER

400ml (1⅔ cups) whole milk

200g (7oz) soft Medjool dates (about 13 dates), pitted

4 large eggs

30g (2 tbsp) unsalted butter, melted, or 2 tbsp vegetable oil, plus extra for greasing

125g (heaping 1 cup) all-purpose flour

2 tbsp cornstarch

Ingredients and recipe continue on the next page

To make the crêpes, heat a large nonstick frying pan over a medium heat. Fill a small bowl with vegetable oil and use a piece of paper towel to wipe a liberal amount of oil onto the frying pan. Use another piece of paper towel to wipe off excess oil. Re-oil the pan between each crêpe using this method.

Using a ladle, stir the batter and then pour a small amount into the frying pan, tilting the pan so the batter covers the base. Cook for around 2 minutes until the edges of the crêpe start to crisp and it releases itself from the pan. Using a spatula, flip it and cook the other side for 30–45 seconds. Once the crêpe is done, move it to a piece of parchment paper to cool.

Stir the batter before you make each crêpe and continue until all of the batter is used: You should end up with around 15–20 crêpes.

To make the filling, whip the cream until thick.

Once the crêpes are completely cool, place a crêpe on your serving plate and spread a little of the whipped cream in a thin layer over the crêpe, leaving a border of about 1cm (½in). Cover with another crêpe and repeat, layering crêpes and cream and finishing with a crêpe for the top of the cake.

Dollop the cake with whipped cream, add a liberal drizzle of the sauce, and garnish with chopped dates.

FOR THE SAUCE

200g (¾ cup plus 2 tbsp) unsalted butter

200g (1 cup) dark brown sugar

2 tbsp white miso

300ml (1¼ cups) heavy cream

FOR THE FILLING

300ml (1¼ cups) heavy cream

FOR THE TOPPING

150ml (½ cup plus 2 tbsp) heavy cream, whipped

10 soft Medjool dates, pitted and roughly chopped

SPECIAL EQUIPMENT: food processor or blender

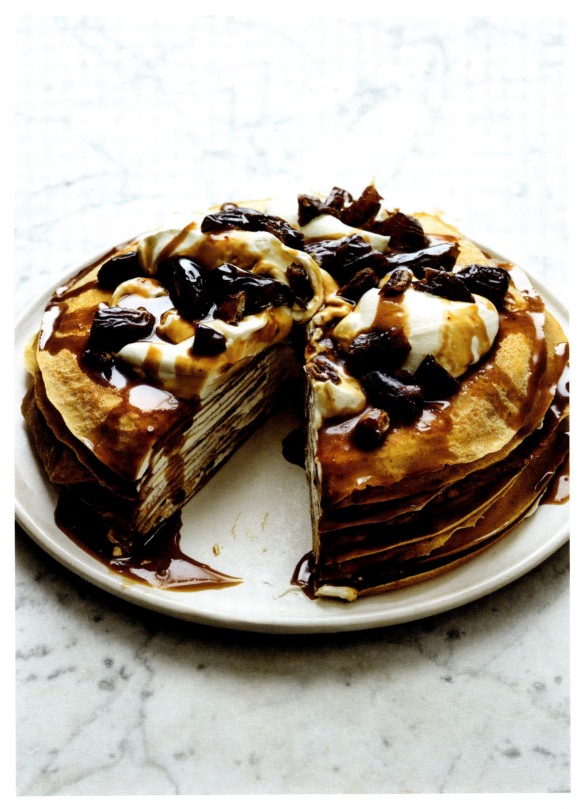

Ricotta & Plum Cheong No-Churn Ice Cream

I always appreciate a simple dessert and it really can't get easier than this no-churn ice cream. Ricotta works really well with the sweet and slightly tangy preserved fruit from cheong. I tried out several varieties of cheong when developing this recipe and plum was my favorite; however, rhubarb and mixed berry will definitely work. This is a great way to use the preserved fruit from cheong, which mixes beautifully with the cream base. The base may seem very sweet, but the sweetened condensed milk makes it easier to scoop as the high sugar levels lower the freezing point of the ice cream.

PREP TIME: 15 MINUTES | FREEZE TIME: 6 HOURS (minimum)

Makes 1.5 liters (1.5 quarts)

- 400ml (1⅔ cups) heavy cream
- 500g (2 cups) ricotta
- 200ml (¾ cup plus 1 tbsp) Plum Cheong (see page 145; prioritize the preserved fruit and top it up with any residual liquid—you want chunks of the preserved fruit throughout the ice cream), plus optional syrup to serve
- one 397-g (14-oz) can condensed milk
- ½ tsp salt
- a few leaves of fresh thyme to serve (optional)

In a large bowl (or electric mixer), whip the heavy cream to soft peaks.

In a separate bowl, mix the ricotta, cheong, condensed milk, and salt. Gently fold this mixture into the whipped cream until evenly mixed.

Put the mixture into freezer-proof containers and freeze for a minimum of 6 hours, or overnight. It should be frozen but soft enough to serve without too much ice crystallization. If it's too hard, take it out of the freezer for 15–20 minutes before serving. Drizzle with plum cheong syrup and decorate with thyme leaves if you like.

This will keep in the freezer for up to 1 month.

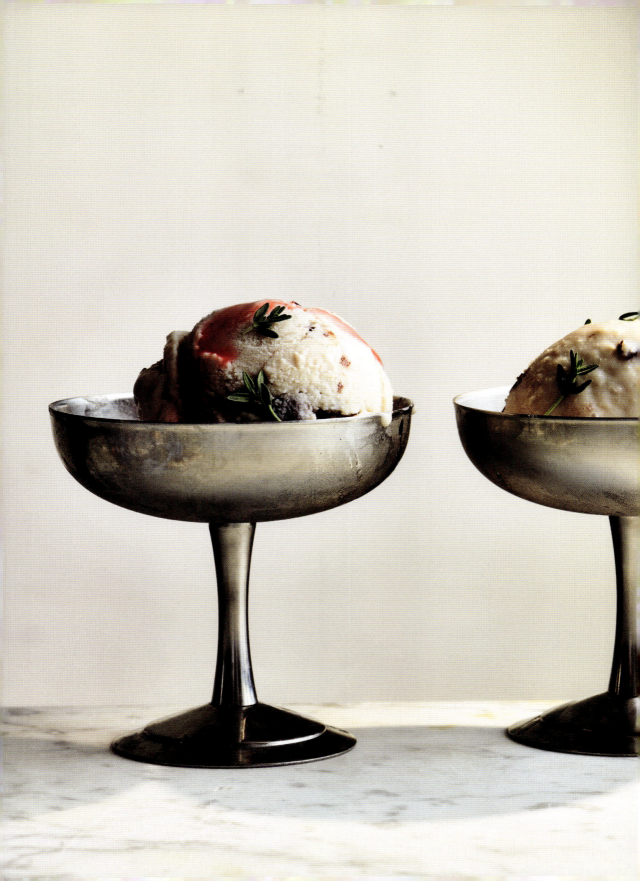

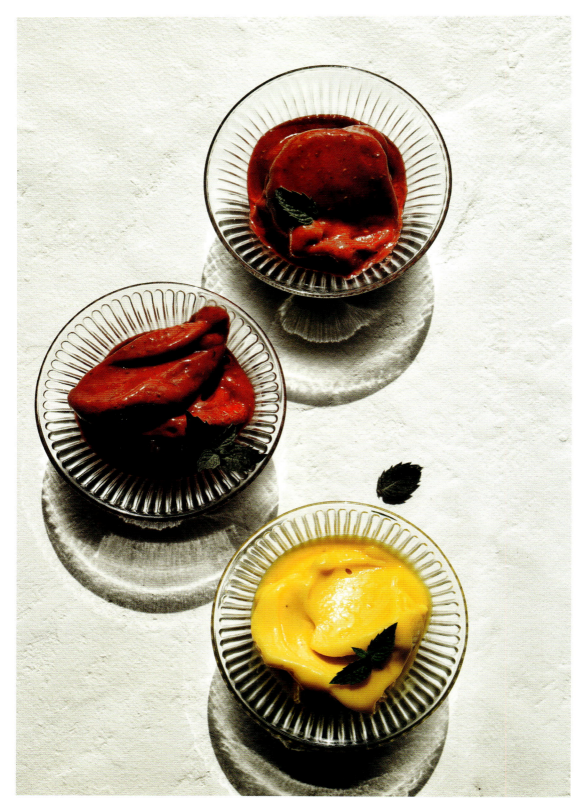

Two-Ingredient Kombucha Sorbet

In the heat of a London summer, I gravitate toward anything icy and everything simple. And so enters this very icy and very simple kombucha sorbet. It does require a powerful food processor or blender to get that sorbet texture; that said, if it ends up as a slushie, it'll be equally good. Any combination of frozen fruit and kombucha will work. Amplify frozen mixed berries with a Frozen Berries & Hibiscus Kombucha or change it up with frozen bananas and Mango & Chili Kombucha (see page 130). Store-bought kombucha will work a treat here. And can you add a shot of your favorite alcohol to make a boozy summer treat? You betcha—it's all about balance.

Stick with 2 parts frozen fruit to 1 part kombucha, though if you want to thin it out, add more kombucha. Depending on the ingredients, you may want to add extra sweetness (from a cheong), acidity (lime or lemon juice), or even a pinch of salt.

PREP TIME: 5 MINUTES

Put the frozen fruit and kombucha into a powerful food processor or blender and blitz at high speed until it reaches your desired consistency.

This does not freeze well and will become too frozen to enjoy as a sorbet, so eat it immediately.

Serves 4

300g (10.5oz) frozen fruit
240ml (1 cup) kombucha

SPECIAL EQUIPMENT: food processor or blender

COCKTAILS

Cucumber Cheong Gimlet

This riff on a gimlet is really just an excuse to celebrate the cucumber, combining cucumber cheong syrup, preserved cucumber, and fresh cucumber. A gimlet is traditionally served in a coupe glass, but if you'd rather make it a long drink, mix it with soda water and call it a day (this is probably no longer a gimlet).

Cucumber cheong has a lot of fun applications in cocktails: Substitute for plain simple syrup for a herbaceous twist or add it to a Pimm's.

PREP TIME: 5 MINUTES

In a large tumbler, muddle the cucumber cheong and the preserved cucumbers (if using). Add the gin, lime juice, and ice to a cocktail shaker and shake until cold. Strain into a coupe glass. Garnish with thinly sliced cucumber.

Serves 1

45ml (3 tbsp) Cucumber Cheong syrup (see page 145)
1 heaping tbsp cheong-preserved cucumbers (if available, otherwise omit)
60ml (¼ cup) gin
30ml (2 tbsp) fresh lime juice
ice
thinly sliced fresh cucumber to garnish

SPECIAL EQUIPMENT: cocktail shaker, coupe glass

Kombucha Citrus Paloma

Perhaps as a result of too much cheap tequila during my youth, it took me a long time to return to this spirit in my adulthood. It was through one of my now-favorite cocktails, the paloma, that I learned to appreciate tequila once again.

Margaritas often steal the limelight of tequila-based cocktails, but grapefruit, further amplified with my kombucha citrus syrup, is just so perfect. But one fermented twist isn't enough, so let's also rim the glass with flaky sea salt laced with kimchi sprinkles.

One note about this cocktail—as the kombucha citrus syrup is 50:50 citrus to sugar, there will definitely be some variance in the sugar content, making it potentially less sweet than if you made a standard simple syrup. I would therefore start off with the recipe below but add more kombucha citrus syrup if needed.

PREP TIME: 5 MINUTES

If necessary, blitz your kimchi sprinkles to a powder and pass them through a fine-mesh strainer. Combine the powdered kimchi sprinkles and sea salt.

To assemble the cocktail, dip the rim of the glass into the kombucha citrus syrup and then into the kimchi and salt mixture.

In a large tumbler, combine the tequila, grapefruit juice, and kombucha citrus syrup. Fill with ice and stir well. Taste and adjust the flavoring and sweetness.

Strain into an ice-filled low tumbler, top up with a splash of soda water, and garnish with a slice of preserved citrus.

Serves 1

1 tsp Kimchi Sprinkles (see page 76)

1 tbsp flaky sea salt

45ml (3 tbsp) Kombucha Citrus Syrup (see page 138)

60ml (¼ cup) tequila

60ml (¼ cup) fresh grapefruit juice

ice

soda water, to taste

preserved citrus slices from the Kombucha Citrus Syrup to garnish

SPECIAL EQUIPMENT: low tumbler

Kimchi Bloody Mary

As with all of the cocktails in this section, the complex flavor here comes from the ferment in question. By first blitzing the ingredients (including the kimchi) and then straining the liquid, you get all of the flavor for this Bloody Mary. While this recipe uses both the brine and the kimchi, it doesn't matter too much if you do not have a ton of kimchi brine on hand. I generally use a cabbage-based kimchi, but the rhubarb and cherry tomato versions (see pages 75 and 66) are also bloody delicious!

PREP TIME: 10 MINUTES

Put all of the ingredients (except the ice and garnishes) into a blender and blitz to extract all of the flavor from the kimchi. Taste and adjust the seasonings.

Strain into an ice-filled highball glass and add your garnishes.

My suggested garnish is a skewer of one piece of kimchi, a slice of Sour Dill Pickle (see page 44), a slice of Quick-Pickled Red Onions (see page 114), a fermented cherry tomato (see page 43), and a lemon wedge. Instead of the skewer, you could go classic and add a celery stick.

Serves 1

60ml (¼ cup) vodka
100ml (¼ cup plus 3 tbsp) tomato juice
25g (2 tbsp plus 2 tsp) kimchi
1 tbsp plus 1 tsp kimchi brine
1 tbsp lemon juice
dash of Tabasco
dash of fish sauce
pinch of celery salt
ice
garnishes of choice (see method)

SPECIAL EQUIPMENT: blender, highball glass

Miso Old Fashioned

Whiskey-based cocktails are my favorite. I didn't want to change much of what I'd consider a perfect cocktail: a sipper, strong, warming, and aromatic. But at this point in the book, you shouldn't be surprised that I like to play with traditions. Here, a subtle saltiness from the miso syrup envelops the mouth, giving an almost buttery taste. So give this miso twist a try—and there'll be extra miso simple syrup on hand, ready to incorporate into other drinks or desserts.

PREP TIME: 10 MINUTES (less if the miso simple syrup is already prepared)

First prepare the miso simple syrup: Put 100ml (¼ cup plus 3 tablespoons) water in a small saucepan over a low heat, add the sugar, and leave until fully dissolved, then remove from the heat and whisk in the miso until fully combined. You can use this syrup as is; however, there will inevitably be bits of miso which will add a cloudiness to your cocktail. I don't mind this cloudiness, but if you prefer a clearer syrup, you can filter it using fine cheesecloth or a coffee filter. Keep the syrup covered in the fridge for up to 1 month.

To assemble the cocktail, fill a large tumbler with ice and add the whiskey, miso simple syrup, and bitters. Stir well, allowing some of the ice to dissolve and cool the drink, then strain into an ice-filled low tumbler. Garnish with orange peel and a maraschino cherry, if you like.

Serves 1

ice
60ml (¼ cup) whiskey
1 tbsp miso simple syrup (see below)
2 dashes of bitters
orange peel to garnish
1 maraschino cherry (optional)

FOR THE MISO SIMPLE SYRUP

100g (½ cup) sugar
20g (1 tbsp plus ½ tsp) white miso

SPECIAL EQUIPMENT: low tumbler

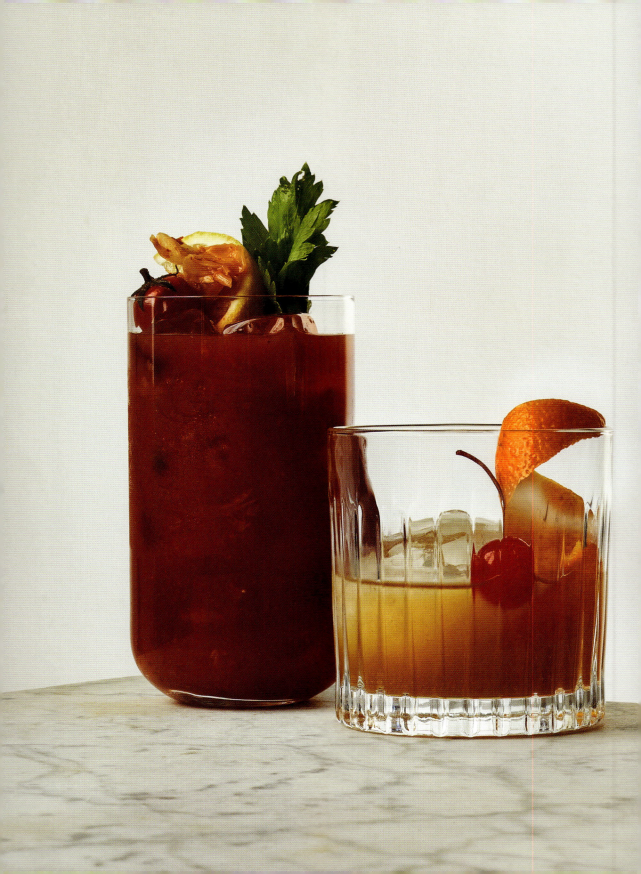

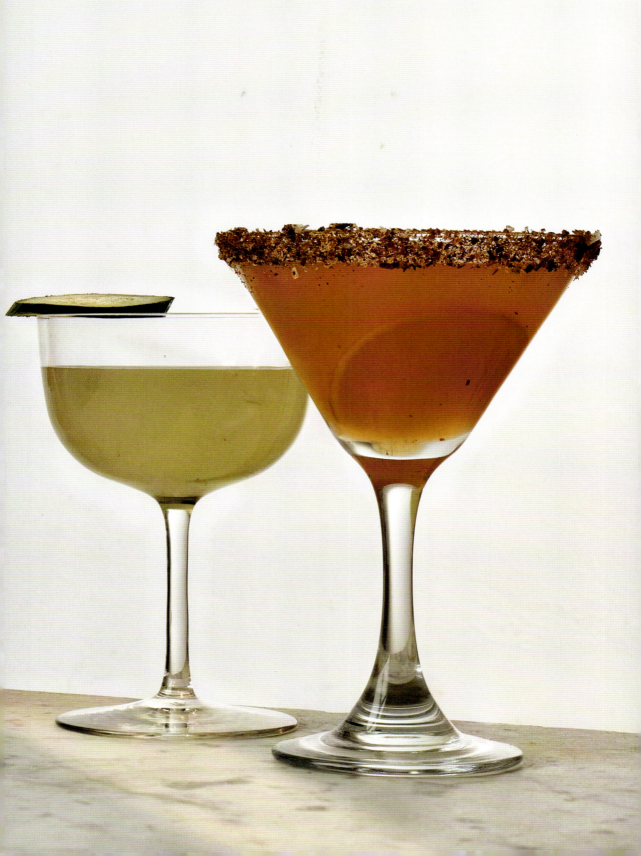

Tomatini

This gin martini is the easiest cocktail, requiring only two ingredients. It really celebrates the humble but complex brine—intensely flavored with tomatoes, and subtle in spice and aromatics from the garlic, onion, and dill.

This is my favorite variation of what I like to call an "any brine" martini: Any fermented brine you have in your kitchen can potentially work. That said, every brine is different—from lactofermented chile sauces to sauerkrauts—so adjust the proportions of gin to brine to your own taste.

PREP TIME: 5 MINUTES

Fill a large tumbler with ice and add the gin and brine. Stir well, then strain into a cold martini glass.

To garnish, go classic with a lemon twist or an olive, or lean into the flavor profile of the brine with a thin slice of tomato and a sprig of fresh dill.

Serves 1

ice
100ml (¼ cup plus 3 tbsp) gin
1 tbsp plus 2 tsp brine from Gazpacho Cherry Tomatoes (see page 43)
garnishes of choice (see method)

SPECIAL EQUIPMENT: martini glass

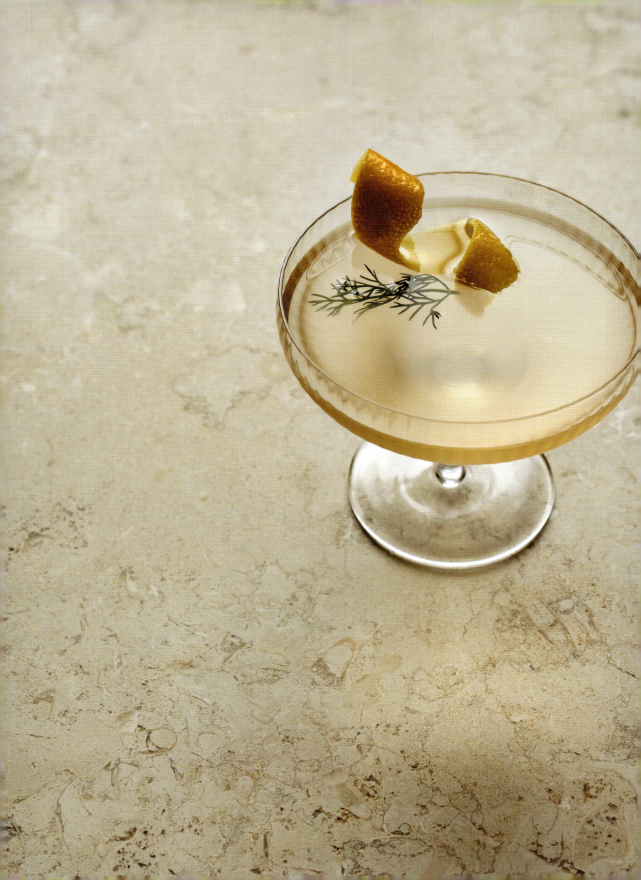

ACKNOWLEDGMENTS

Thank you to the team behind this book, whose steadfast belief in me made this dream a reality.

To my publisher, Lizzy Gray, for your expertise and kindness, and for trusting me with autonomy with this debut book. To my managing editor, Martha Burley, whose seamless organization knows no bounds and whose collaborative support made this process a joy. To my copy editors and proofreaders, Maggie Ramsay and Laura Nickoll, whose wordsmithery and attention to detail provided consistency and flow.

To my creative team, namely Claire Rochford, Dan Jones, and Anna Wilkins, whose aesthetics, vision, and sheer skill (and music knowledge) blew me away. To my food stylist, Katy McClelland, and her team (Nicola Roberts, Lauren Wall, and Melanie McIntosh), for not only making these recipes prettier than I ever could, but also being so much fun in the kitchen. I'm also very pleased that the shoot has inspired many of you to start your own fermentation journeys.

And to my literary agent, Sabhbh Curran, for challenging me to hone my voice and finesse the stories I endeavor to tell.

Team, I am in awe of your professionalism, artistic prowess, and ability to breathe such vibrant life into a concept. I couldn't have been happier working with you all and feel very lucky to have learned so much from each and every one of you. Writing and developing a cookbook can be a rather solitary exercise, and working with you all made the journey so worth it.

Thank you to my teachers, both near and far, whose knowledge has been a springboard for creativity and a collaborative source for advice and collective learning as I've jumped into the many rabbit holes that connected to fermentation and preservation at home. There are many people to name, however, those at the front of my mind are Kirsten Shockey, Rich Shih, and Jeremy Umansky, whose books gave me the confidence to create and explore; Payal Shah, whose passion for fermentation was a lifeline for me during the pandemic; and Melanie McIntosh, who has been a friend throughout my entire food journey and from whom I've learned so much. Fermentation is symbolic of even larger things in our lives: It's transformative and I'm always amazed at how this approach to food and flavor can cultivate and develop a global sense of community for which I'm truly grateful.

Thank you to my community of fermentation friends across the globe, to those rediscovering family traditions and most importantly, the memories they carry. It's been incredibly rewarding to hear your stories of common ground unearthed through flavor, but also so inspiring to witness your own sparks of creation in your home kitchens. While overstated, it's absolutely true that none of this would have been possible without your engagement so a genuine and heartfelt thank you.

Thank you to my family, who unbeknownst to them, created a home where passions could be pursued and creativity cultivated, and instilled in me such a strong sense of family and identity which has been a driving force in everything I do. To my sister, Emiko, who, as a deft canner and jam maker, was arguably my first influence in appreciating the beauty and self-reliance in the humble glass jar. To my parents, Joyce and Rick, for your never-ending love, patience, and encouragement—especially when my path diverged from one of familiarity or comfort. It's been quite the ride as I've gone through the trials and tribulations of growing up and finding my own voice. And I can say with great confidence that my interests and accomplishments are a product of you.

And thank you to Will, my biggest advocate, constructive critic, earliest proofreader, chief taste tester, and the reason I strive to be a better cook. You've always encouraged me to explore and invest in my passions and have been my cheerleader, from near and far. You've allowed me to grow—and have shown patience and understanding with the ever-increasing number of jars in the house. Cooking is my love language, as it is for many, and the ability to feed you with food—fermented and otherwise—that culminates in and is a reflection of who I am is the greatest honor.

INDEX

A
aerobic processes 135
aioli, miso 208, **209**
amino (miso-like) paste 83, 85
anaerobic processes 15, 27
apple 50, 55, 58, 69
apple cider vinegar 107, 109, 111, 114, 116, 120–1, 194
arancini, kimchi 174–5, **176–7**
arugula & fennel miso Caesar 194
Aspergillus oryzae 81

B
bacon, leek & kimchi quiche 225–6, **227**
bacteria 15, 20, 26, 29, 32, 107, 135–7, 150–1
bean(s) 172, 232
　green mean bean miso soup with curried crispy lima beans 198, **199**
　spicy green beans **110**, 111
béchamel 206, **207**, 229, **231**
beef, miso short rib birria tacos with kimchi guacamole & umami slaw 233–4, **235**
beet miso with cumin & allspice 98–9, **100**
berries
　blueberry & rosemary kombucha 131, **132**
　frozen berries & hibiscus kombucha 130, **132**
　mixed berry cheong 144, **146**, 242
　preserved rhubarb & mixed berry pound cake 242, **243**
bhaji, kimchi onion 168–9, **170–1**
biscuits, kimchi & cheddar 180, **182–3**
blondies **238**, 239
Bloody Mary, kimchi 256, **258**
blueberry & rosemary kombucha 131, **132**
botulism 20

brine 63, 107, 174–5
　dry brining 26, 28–9, **30–1**
　keeping ferments below 15–16, **22–3**, 27–8, 32, 40, 86, 143
　uses for 27, 63, 153
　wet brining 26–7, 32, **34–5**
brussels sprouts 223–4
　Brussels sprout & cranberry kimchi **68**, 69
bubbling 15, 27, 29, 32, 128
burping containers 15, 27, 29, 32, 128, 136
butter
　gochujang 200–1
　miso 178, **179**
butternut, broccoli & lentils with charred leek & miso tahini yogurt 188–90, **189**

C
cabbage 16, 20, 26, 36, 47, 54–5, 58, 71, 151
Caesar dressing, miso 194, 208
cakes 242, **243**, 247–8, **249**
caponata, kimchi 195
carbon dioxide 15, 29, 32, 128, 136
carrot 38, 54–5, 58, 62–3, 70, 223–4
　chipotle & carrot sauerkraut 51
　kombucha-pickled carrot & daikon 117, **119**, 208
cheddar 206, 225–6
　kimchi & cheddar biscuits 180, **182–3**
cheese 163, 174–5, 194, 208, 250
　see also cheddar; feta
cheong 142–7
　cheong 101 143
　cheong kombucha 131
　cucumber cheong 145, **146**, 254
　cucumber cheong gimlet 254, **259**

mixed berry cheong 144, **146**, 242
plum cheong 145, **147**
rhubarb cheong 144, **146**, 242, 245
rhubarb cheong pavlova **244**, 245
ricotta & plum cheong no-churn ice cream 250, **251**
chicken
　chicken kimchi masala 214, **215**
　kimchi-brined fried chicken with gochujang hot honey crumpets 218–19, **220–1**
　leftover (Sunday) roast chicken miso noodle soup **222**, 223–4
　miso ginger chicken orzo 216–17
chickpea & sauerkraut salad 191
chile 104, 178
　chile, orange & coriander sauerkraut **46**, 47
　chili crisp balsamic roasted tomatoes 192, **193**
　and lactofermentation 36, 41, 43–5, 47–8
　mango & chili kombucha 130, **132**
　pickled pears with thyme, chile & coriander 121, **123**
　and pickles 109, 111–12, 116–17, 121
　pineapple & Scotch bonnet hot sauce **48**, 49
　quick-pickled kombucha chiles 112, **113**
　see also gochugaru chili
chimichurri paste, koji 104, **105**
chipotle & carrot sauerkraut 51
chocolate chip blondies **238**, 239
chutneys 168–9, **170–1**, 181, **182–3**

cilantro (fresh) 41, 70, 178,
    185, 214
  cilantro & mint miso chutney
    168–9, **170–1**
citrus fruit 104
  citrus kombucha cookies
    240, **241**
  citrus miso salmon &
    edamame rice **210**, 211
  see also kombucha citrus
    syrup
cleanliness 20–1
cocktails 254–60
Comté arancini 174–5, **176–7**
containers 17–19
cookies, citrus kombucha
    240, **241**
coriander (seed) 47, 121
zucchini 195
  zucchini bread & butter
    pickles **108**, 109, 205
  umami zucchini 172, **173**
cranberry & Brussels sprout
    kimchi **68**, 69
cream 245, 247–8, 250
crêpe cake 247–8, **249**
croutons 194
crudités, fermented 38, **39**
crumpets, hot honey 218–19,
    220–1
cucumber 44, 162
  crunchy soy sauce cucumbers
    116, **118**
  cucumber cheong 145, **146**,
    254
  cucumber cheong gimlet
    254, **259**
  cucumber snake-cut kimchi
    62–3, **64–5**
curries 36, 185, 198, 202, 214

D

date & miso sticky toffee crêpe
    cake 247–8, **249**
dehydrating ferments 76–7
desserts 236–53
dill 43
  dill yogurt 160–1
  sour dill pickles 44, 185
dip, nuoc cham 205
discoloration 16, 27
dressings **184**, 185, 208

E

edamame rice **210**, 211
eggplant 195, 228–9
environmental factors 21
equipment 17–19

F

fennel
  fennel, apple & caraway
    sauerkraut 50
  fennel & arugula miso Caesar
    with charred miso Parm
    croutons 194
  fennel & turmeric kimchi 71,
    72–3
  kimchi & fennel sausage rolls
    166, 167
fermentation signs 15, 29, 32
fermentation weights 15, 28, 32,
    85, 142–3
ferments 24–147, 150–1
feta 178, 191, 197, 233–4
  kimchi & feta spanakopita
    200–1
  phyllo pastry, spanakopita
    200–1
fish
  citrus miso salmon &
    edamame rice **210**, 211
  fried fish sandwich with
    pickles & miso aioli 208, **209**
  miso fishermen's pie 206, **207**
  sweet pickle tuna summer
    rolls **204**, 205
fruit
  cut fruit with kombucha citrus
    syrup & kimchi sprinkles
    246
  pickled fruit tart with goat
    cheese 163, **164–5**
  see also specific fruit

G

garlic misozuke 97
gazpacho cherry tomatoes **42**,
    43, 260
  fermented gazpacho 162
gimlet, cucumber cheong
    254, **259**
gin-based cocktails 254, 260
ginger (fresh root)
  ginger, honey & lemon
    kombucha 131, 132

ginger miso **101**, 102–3
  miso ginger chicken orzo
    216–17
  pickled grapes with ginger &
    allspice 121, **122**
glazes 240, **241**
goat cheese with pickled fruit
    tart 163, **164–5**
gochugaru chili 52–3, 212, 214
  ferments 55, 58, 60, 62–3, 66,
    69–70, 75
gochujang 174–5
  gochujang butter 200–1
  gochujang hot honey 218–19
grape(s), pickled 121, **122**
Greek-style yogurt 242
  miso tahini yogurt 188–90, **189**
guacamole, kimchi 233–4, **235**
gut microbiome 11

H

harissa & kimchi shakshuka
    196, 197
hibiscus & frozen berries
    kombucha 130, **132**
hissing 15, 27
honey 135
  ginger, honey & lemon
    kombucha 131, **132**
  gochujang hot honey 218–19
  hot honey crumpets 218–19,
    220–1
hot sauces 19, 45, 48, **49**
hummus, miso 172, **173**

I

ice cream 250, **251**
ingredients 20
  see also specific ingredients
iodine 20

J

jun 135

K

kimchi 16, 26, 52–77, 70, 151
  bacon, leek & kimchi quiche
    225–6, **227**
  Brussels sprout & cranberry
    kimchi **68**, 69
  cherry tomato kimchi 66, **67**
  chicken kimchi masala 214,
    215

kimchi (*continued*)
  corner store kimchi 58, **59**
  cucumber snake-cut
    kimchi 62–3, **64–5**
  fennel & turmeric kimchi
    71, **72–3**
  fermentation temperature
    52, 53
  kimchi 101 54–5, **56–7**
  kimchi & cheddar biscuits
    180, **182–3**
  kimchi & fennel sausage rolls
    166, 167
  kimchi & feta spanakopita
    with gochujang butter 200–1
  kimchi & harissa shakshuka
    196, 197
  kimchi Bloody Mary 256, **258**
  kimchi caponata 195
  kimchi fried rice Comté
    arancini 174–5, **176–7**
  kimchi guacamole 233–4, **235**
  kimchi onion bhaji with
    cilantro & mint miso chutney
    168–9, **170–1**
  kimchi sprinkles 76–7, **78–9**,
    178, 205, 246, 255
  kimchi-brined fried chicken
    with gochujang hot honey
    crumpets 218–19, **220–1**
  pickle platters 152
  red onion & kimchi chutney,
    two ways 181, **182–3**
  rhubarb kimchi **74**, 75
  ten-minute miso peanut
    butter kimchi noodles 212,
    213
  watermelon rind kimchi 60, **61**
koji 81, 88, 90–1, 95–6, 98–9,
  102–3
  koji chimichurri paste 104, **105**
  koji starters 81, 84, 85
kombucha 19, 124–39, **125**
  blueberry & rosemary
    kombucha 131, **132**
  carbonation 128, 135–6
  cheong kombucha 131
  citrus kombucha cookies
    240, **241**
  continuous brewing 136
  decanting 128
  effervescence 124, 126, 128,
    135–6

first fermentation 126–8, 135–7
frozen berries & hibiscus
  kombucha 130, **132**
ginger, honey & lemon
  kombucha 131, **132**
kombucha 101 127–8, **129**
kombucha citrus paloma
  255, **259**
kombucha citrus syrup 66,
  138–9, **140–1**, 188–90, 205,
  211, 240, 246, 255
kombucha-pickled carrot
  & daikon 117, **119**, 208
mango & chili kombucha
  130, **132**
quick-pickled kombucha
  chiles 112, **113**
SCOBY (starter/pellicle)
  124–8, **124**, 134–7
secondary fermentation
  126–8, 135–7
sour 137
temperature 127–8, 135
two-ingredient kombucha
  sorbet **252**, 253

L

lactic acid 15, 26
lactobacillus 15, 26
lactofermentation 15–17, 21,
  26–51, 152
lamb, nasu dengaku moussaka
  228–9, **231**
latkes, sauerkraut 160–1
leek 232
  bacon, leek & kimchi quiche
    225–6, **227**
  charred leek 188–90, **189**
legumes 81, 85, 88
  see also specific legumes
lemon, ginger & honey
  kombucha 131, **132**
lettuce 205, 208
lids, breathable 135

M

mains 188–234
mango & chili kombucha 130,
  132
marinades 214, **215**
masala, chicken kimchi 214, **215**
massaging vegetables 26, 28
metals 135

mint (fresh) 41, 185, 245
  cilantro & mint miso chutney
    168–9, **170–1**
miso 69, 80–104, 151, 153
  beet miso with cumin
    & allspice 98–9, **100**
  decanting 86
  ginger miso **101**, 102–3
  miso aioli 208, **209**
  miso butter corn ribs elote
    178, **179**
  pumpkin miso **94**, 95–6
  timings 82
  unpasteurised 85, 90–1
miso (red) 88–91, 97, 151, 202,
  228–9
  cilantro & mint miso chutney
    168–9, **170–1**
  citrus miso salmon **210**, 211
  garlic misozuke 97
  green mean bean miso soup
    198, **199**
  leftover (Sunday) roast
    chicken miso noodle soup
    222, 223–4
  miso Caesar dressing 194, 208
  miso fishermen's pie 206, **207**
  miso ginger chicken orzo
    216–17
  miso hummus 172, **173**
  miso pesto pasta salad with
    chili crisp balsamic roasted
    tomatoes 192, **193**
  miso short rib birria tacos
    with kimchi guacamole &
    umami slaw 233–4, **235**
  miso tahini yogurt 188–90, **189**
  red miso 101 84–6
  ten-minute miso peanut
    butter kimchi noodles 212,
    213
miso (white) 88–91, **89**, 151, 172,
  234
  citrus miso salmon &
    edamame rice **210**, 211
  citrus miso sauce 211
  date & miso sticky toffee
    crêpe cake 247–8, **249**
  miso hummus with umami
    zucchini & pine nuts 172, **173**
  miso old fashioned 257, **258**
  miso praline sesame pecans
    186, 236, **237**

miso simple syrup 257
miso tahini chocolate chip blondies **238**, 239
miso tahini yogurt 188–90, **189**
misozuke, garlic 97
mold 15–16, 19, 21, 27, 32, 86, 135
morkovcha 70

N

nasu dengaku moussaka 228–9, **230–1**
noodles 212, **213**, **222**, 223–4
nuoc cham dip 205

O

old fashioned, miso 257, **258**
onion
  ferments 36, 43, 45, 48, 55, 109, 114
  kimchi onion bhaji 168–9, **170–1**
  quick-pickled red onions 114, **115**
  red onion & kimchi chutney 181, **182–3**orange 75
  chile, orange & coriander sauerkraut **46**, 47
orzo, miso ginger chicken 216–17
oxidation 16, 27, 147
oxygen 15–16, 19, 21, 86, 135, 143

P

paloma, kombucha citrus 255, **259**
panko bread crumbs 174–5, 208
parsley (fresh) 104, 186, 190, 197, 232
pasta 192, **193**, 216–17
pasteurization 150
pastry 225–6, **227**
  see also phyllo pastry; puff pastry (ready-rolled)
pavlova, rhubarb cheong **244**, 245
peanut 169
  ten-minute miso peanut butter kimchi noodles 212, **213**
pear
  pickled pear vinaigrette 186, **187**

pickled pears with thyme, chile & coriander 121, **123**
pecan, miso praline sesame 236, **237**
pesto, miso 192, **193**
pickle packers 19
pickles 106–21
  cooking with 150–1
  zucchini bread & butter pickles **108**, 109, 205
  crunchy soy sauce cucumbers 116, **118**
  curried pickle smashed potato salad **184**, 185
  fried fish sandwich with pickles & miso aioli 208, **209**
  kombucha-pickled carrot & daikon 117, **119**, 208
  pickle platters 152–3, **154–5**
  pickled fruit tart with goat cheese 163, **164–5**
  pickled fruit, three ways 120–1, **122–3**
  pickled grapes with ginger & allspice 121, **122**
  pickled pear vinaigrette 186, **187**
  pickled pears with thyme, chile & coriander 121, **123**
  pickled plums with star anise & pink peppercorns 120, **123**
  quick-pickled kombucha chiles 112, **113**
  quick-pickled red onions 114, **115**
  sour dill pickles 44
  spicy green beans **110**, 111
  sweet pickle tuna summer rolls **204**, 205
pie, miso fishermen's 206, **207**
pineapple & Scotch bonnet hot sauce 48, **49**
plum
  pickled plums with star anise & pink peppercorns 120, **123**
  plum cheong 145, **147**
  ricotta & plum cheong no-churn ice cream 250, **251**
potato 160–1, 206
  curried pickle smashed potato salad **184**, 185
praline, miso praline sesame pecans 186, 236, **237**

puff pastry (ready-rolled) 163, **164–5**, **166**, 167
pumpkin miso **94**, 95–6

Q

quiche 225–6, **227**

R

radish (daikon) (mooli) 54–5
  kombucha pickled carrot & daikon 117, **119**, 208
refrigeration 29, 32, 53, 86, 128
rhubarb
  preserved rhubarb & mixed berry pound cake 242, **243**
  rhubarb cheong 144, **146**, 242, 245
  rhubarb cheong pavlova **244**, 245
  rhubarb kimchi **74**, 75
rice
  edamame rice **210**, 211
  kimchi fried rice Comté arancini 174–5, **176–7**
  rice porridge 54–5
ricotta & plum cheong no-churn ice cream 250, **251**

S

salads **184**, 185–6, **187**, 191–2, **193**, 194
salmon, citrus miso salmon & edamame rice **210**, 211
salt 20–1, 107
  and dry brining 26, 28
  measurement 17
  and miso 82, 84, 88, 90–1, 95–6, 98–9, 102–3
  and wet brining 27, 32
sandwich, fried fish 208, **209**
sauces
  béchamel 206, **207**, 229, **231**
  citrus miso **210**, 211
  everyday hot 45
  miso butter 178, **179**
  nuoc cham dipping 205
  pineapple & Scotch bonnet hot 48, **49**
sauerkraut 20, 21, 26, 151
  chickpea & sauerkraut salad 191
  chile, orange & coriander sauerkraut **46**, 47

sauerkraut (*continued*)
  chipotle & carrot sauerkraut 51
  dry brining 26
  fennel, apple & caraway sauerkraut 50
  garam masala sauerkraut 36, 37
  kraut & sausage soup with sour cream & parsley 232
  sauercaccia 156–7, **157**, **158–9**
  sauerkraut latkes with dill yogurt 160–1
sausage meat
  kimchi & fennel sausage rolls **166**, 167
  kraut & sausage soup with sour cream & parsley 232
seasonality 10, 60, 69, 75, 95, 106
sesame seed 62–3, 174–5
  black 60, 167, 186, 200–1, 211, 219, 236
  miso praline sesame pecans 186, 236, **237**
  white 70, 186, 192, 219, 236
shakshuka, kimchi & harissa **196**, 197
simple syrup, miso 257
slaw, umami 233–4, **235**
sorbet, kombucha **252**, 253
soups 198, **199**, **222**, 223–4, 232
soy sauce 178, 202
  crunchy soy sauce cucumbers 116, **118**
soybean(s) 81, 84–5, 88, 90–1, **210**, 211
spanakopita, kimchi & feta 200–1
spinach 200–1, 223–4
green onion 205–6, 225–6
  ferments 54–5, 58, 62–3, 66, 71, 75, 211
starters 152–86
sugar
  and cheong 142–3, 144–5
  and kombucha 126–8, 134–7, 139
  and pickles 107, 109, 111–12, 114, 116–17, 120–1
summer rolls **204**, 205
sunlight 21, 32

sweetcorn, miso butter corn ribs elote 178, **179**
syrups *see* cheong; kombucha citrus syrup

T
tacos 233–4, **235**
tahini 172
  miso tahini chocolate chip blondies **238**, 239
  miso tahini yogurt 188–90, **189**
tamari, pooling 86
tart, pickled fruit 163, **164–5**
tasting ferments 16, 27
tea, fermented *see* kombucha
temperature 21, 27, 29, 32, 52–3, 127–8, 135
tequila-based cocktails 255
toffee crêpe cake 247–8, **249**
tomatini 260, **261**
tomato 195, 197, 256
  cherry tomato kimchi 66, **67**
  chili crisp balsamic roasted tomatoes 192, **193**
  gazpacho cherry tomatoes **42**, 43, 162, 260
tsukemono (Japanese pickles) 97
tuna, sweet pickle tuna summer rolls **204**, 205

U
umeshu (plum wine) 145

V
vinaigrette 186, **187**
vinegars 107, 192
  see also apple cider vinegar
vodka-based cocktails 256

W
watermelon rind kimchi 60, **61**
weights and measures 17, 28, 32
whiskey-based cocktails 257

Y
yeast 127–8, 135–7, 143, 156–7
  kahm 21, **22**, 40
  unwanted 15, 19, 21, **22**, 27, 32, 40, 86
yogurt 169, 185, 190, 214, 234, 245

dill yogurt 160–1
  see also Greek-style yogurt

Z
zero-waste green paste 22–3, **23**, 40–1, 202

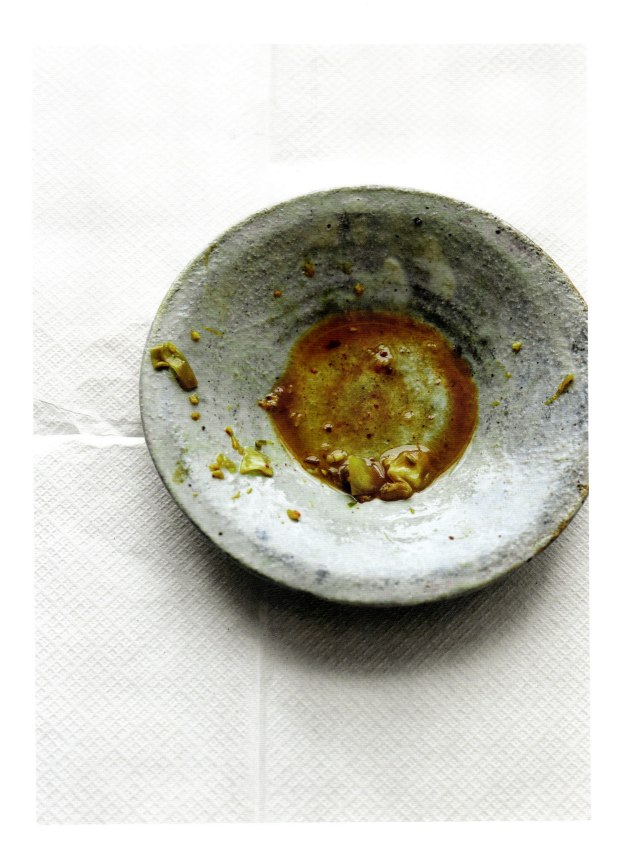

ABOUT KENJI

Kenji Morimoto is a content creator and food writer based in London. As a fourth-generation Japanese American, his cultural identity has always been grounded in food. As a child, he was in charge of making tsukemono (Japanese pickles) for family gatherings, learning from and surrounded by elders recreating the flavors of home. In 2020, he started his Instagram @kenjcooks to document his interest in fermentation and connecting the dots between diasporic traditions and his own. Since then, he's cooked in kitchens in Poland, held residencies in London restaurants, including Ottolenghi's ROVI, led fermentation and Japanese-focused supper clubs in London, taught workshops on koji and kimchi, and collaborated with the Ottolenghi Test Kitchen and the nutrition app Zoe. He has been published in *Delicious*, *Guardian Feast*, and *Waitrose Food* publications, and spoken on panels at the British Library on themes of community, food, and immigrant narratives. In 2023, he was a finalist for the BBC Food & Farming Digital Creator of the Year Award.

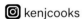 kenjcooks

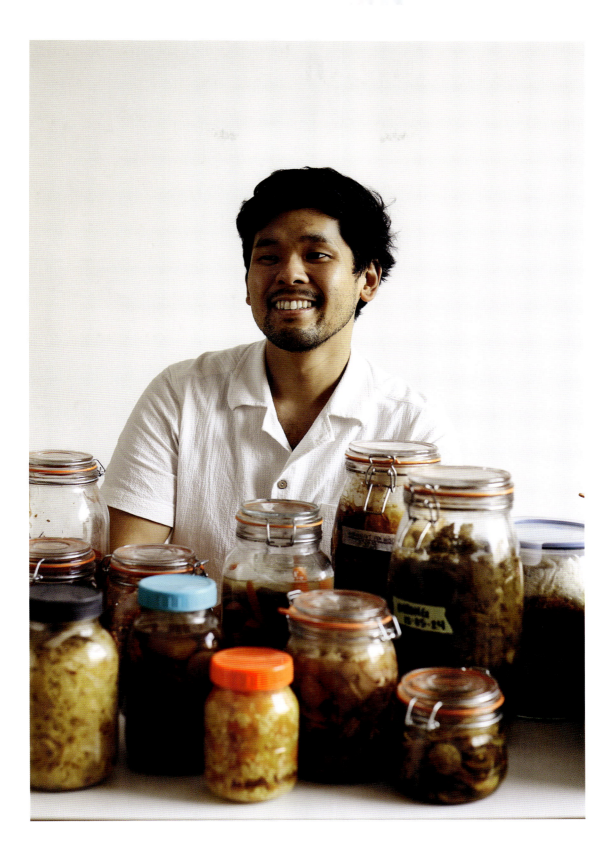

FERMENT: *Simple Recipes from My Multicultural Kitchen*
Copyright © 2025 by Kenji Morimoto
Photographs, including author photograph, copyright © 2025 by Dan Jones

Originally published in the UK by One Boat, an imprint of Pan Macmillan, part of Macmillan Publishers International Limited. First published in North America in revised form by The Experiment, LLC.

All rights reserved. Except for brief passages quoted in newspaper, magazine, radio, television, or online reviews, no portion of this book may be reproduced, distributed, or transmitted in any form or by any means, electronic or mechanical, including photocopying, recording, or information storage or retrieval system, without the prior written permission of the publisher.

The Experiment, LLC
220 East 23rd Street, Suite 600
New York, NY 10010-4658
theexperimentpublishing.com

This book contains the opinions and ideas of its author. It is intended to provide helpful and informative material on the subjects addressed in the book. It is sold with the understanding that the author and publisher are not engaged in rendering medical, health, or any other kind of personal professional services in the book. The author and publisher specifically disclaim all responsibility for any liability, loss, or risk—personal or otherwise—that is incurred as a consequence, directly or indirectly, of the use and application of any of the contents of this book.

THE EXPERIMENT and its colophon are registered trademarks of The Experiment, LLC. Many of the designations used by manufacturers and sellers to distinguish their products are claimed as trademarks. Where those designations appear in this book and The Experiment was aware of a trademark claim, the designations have been capitalized.

The Experiment's books are available at special discounts when purchased in bulk for premiums and sales promotions as well as for fund-raising or educational use. For details, contact us at info@theexperimentpublishing.com.

Library of Congress Cataloging-in-Publication Data

Names: Morimoto, Kenji author
Title: Ferment : simple recipes from my multicultural kitchen / Kenji
  Morimoto.
Description: New York : The Experiment, [2025] | Includes index.
Identifiers: LCCN 2025014730 (print) | LCCN 2025014731 (ebook) | ISBN
  9798893030778 | ISBN 9798893030785 ebook
Subjects: LCSH: Cooking (Fermented foods) | Fermented foods | Fermentation
  | LCGFT: Cookbooks
Classification: LCC TX827.5 .M675 2025 (print) | LCC TX827.5 (ebook) |
  DDC 641.6/163--dc23/eng/20250408
LC record available at https://lccn.loc.gov/2025014730
LC ebook record available at https://lccn.loc.gov/2025014731

ISBN 979-8-89303-077-8
Ebook ISBN 979-8-89303-078-5

Cover and text design by Beth Bugler, based on design by Claire Rochford
Cover illustration by Claire Rochford
Food and prop styling by Katy McClelland, Lauren Wall, Nicola Roberts, Melanie McIntosh, and Anna Wilkins

Manufactured in China

First printing September 2025
10 9 8 7 6 5 4 3 2 1

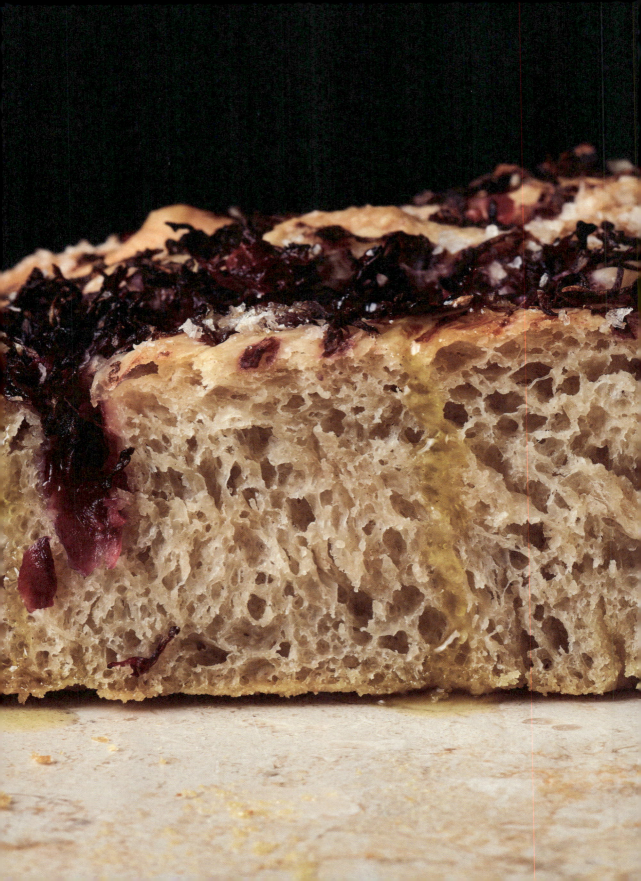

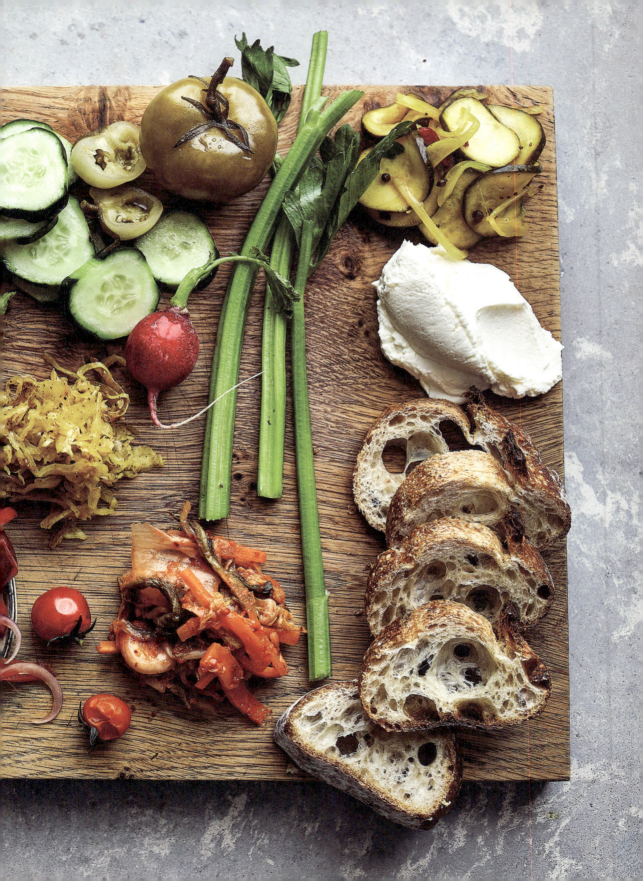